Ergebnisse der Anatomie und Entwicklungsgeschichte
Advances in Anatomy, Embryology and Cell Biology
Revues d'anatomie et de morphologie expérimentale

Springer-Verlag · Berlin · Heidelberg · New York

This journal publishes reviews and critical articles covering the entire field of normal anatomy (cytology, histology, cyto- and histochemistry, electron microscopy, macroscopy, experimental morphology and embryology and comparative anatomy). Papers dealing with anthropology and clinical morphology will also be accepted with the aim of encouraging co-operation between anatomy and related disciplines.

Papers, which may be in English, French or German, are normally commissioned, but original papers and communications may be submitted and will be considered so long as they deal with a subject comprehensively and meet the requirements of the Ergebnisse.

For speed of publication and breadth of distribution, this journal appears in single issues which can be purchased separately; 6 issues constitute one volume.

It is a fundamental condition that manuscripts submitted should not have been published elsewhere, in this or any other country, and the author must undertake not to publish elsewhere at a later date.

25 copies of each paper are supplied free of charge.

Les résultats publient des sommaires et des articles critiques concernant l'ensemble du domaine de l'anatomie normale (cytologie, histologie, cyto et histochimie, microscopie électronique, macroscopie, morphologie expérimentale, embryologie et anatomie comparée. Seront publiés en outre les articles traitant de l'anthropologie et de la morphologie clinique, en vue d'encourager la collaboration entre l'anatomie et les disciplines voisines.

Seront publiés en priorité les articles expressément demandés nous tiendrons toutefois compte des articles qui nous seront envoyés dans la mesure où ils traitent d'un sujet dans son ensemble et correspondent aux standards des «Résultats». Les publications seront faites en langues anglaise, allemande et française.

Dans l'intérêt d'une publication rapide et d'une large diffusion les travaux publiés paraitront dans des cahiers individuels, diffusés séparément: 6 cahiers forment un volume.

En principe, seuls les manuscrits qui n'ont encore été publiés ni dans le pays d'origine ni à l'étranger peuvent nous être soumis. L'auteur d'engage en outre à ne pas les publier ailleurs ultérieurement.

Les auteurs recevront 25 exemplaires gratuits de leur publication.

Die Ergebnisse dienen der Veröffentlichung zusammenfassender und kritischer Artikel aus dem Gesamtgebiet der normalen Anatomie (Cytologie, Histologie, Cyto- und Histochemie, Elektronenmikroskopie, Makroskopie, experimentelle Morphologie und Embryologie und vergleichende Anatomie). Aufgenommen werden ferner Arbeiten anthropologischen und morphologisch-klinischen Inhaltes, mit dem Ziel die Zusammenarbeit zwischen Anatomie und Nachbardisziplinen zu fördern.

Zur Veröffentlichung gelangen in erster Linie angeforderte Manuskripte, jedoch werden auch eingesandte Arbeiten und Originalmitteilungen berücksichtigt, sofern sie ein Gebiet umfassend abhandeln und den Anforderungen der „Ergebnisse" genügen. Die Veröffentlichungen erfolgen in englischer, deutscher oder französischer Sprache.

Die Arbeiten erscheinen im Interesse einer raschen Veröffentlichung und einer weiten Verbreitung als einzeln berechnete Hefte; je 6 Hefte bilden einen Band.

Grundsätzlich dürfen nur Manuskripte eingesandt werden, die vorher weder im Inland noch im Ausland veröffentlicht worden sind. Der Autor verpflichtet sich, sie auch nachträglich nicht an anderen Stellen zu publizieren.

Die Mitarbeiter erhalten von ihren Arbeiten zusammen 25 Freiexemplare.

Manuscripts should be addressed to/Envoyer les manuscrits à/Manuskripte sind zu senden an:

Prof. Dr. A. BRODAL, Universitetet i Oslo, Anatomisk Institutt, Karl Johans Gate 47 (Domus Media), Oslo 1/Norwegen.

Prof. W. HILD, Department of Anatomy, The University of Texas Medical Branch, Galveston, Texas 77550 (USA).

Prof. Dr. R. ORTMANN, Anatomisches Institut der Universität, 5 Köln-Lindenthal, Lindenburg.

Prof. Dr. T.H. SCHIEBLER, Anatomisches Institut der Universität, Koellikerstraße 6, 87 Würzburg.

Prof. Dr. G. TÖNDURY, Direktion der Anatomie, Gloriastraße 19, CH-8006 Zürich.

Prof. Dr. E. WOLFF, Collège de France, Laboratoire d'Embryologie Expérimentale, 49 bis Avenue de la belle Gabrielle, Nogent-sur-Marne 94/France.

Ergebnisse der Anatomie und Entwicklungsgeschichte
Advances in Anatomy, Embryology and Cell Biology
Revues d'anatomie et de morphologie expérimentale

42 · 4

Editores

A. Brodal, Oslo · W. Hild, Galveston · R. Ortmann, Köln
T. H. Schiebler, Würzburg · G. Töndury, Zürich · E. Wolff, Paris

Mark E. Molliver and Hendrik Van der Loos

The Ontogenesis of Cortical Circuitry: The Spatial Distribution of Synapses in Somesthetic Cortex of Newborn Dog

With 64 Figures

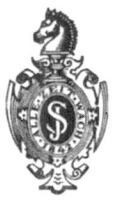

Springer-Verlag Berlin Heidelberg New York 1970

Mark E. Molliver, M. D., and Hendrik Van der Loos, M. D.
Department of Anatomy
The Johns Hopkins University, School of Medicine
Baltimore, Maryland 21205 (USA)

ISBN 978-3-540-04797-1   ISBN 978-3-642-51631-3 (eBook)
DOI 10.1007/978-3-642-51631-3

Contents

Introduction

The ontogenesis of cortical circuitry is the subject of the investigation reported in this paper[1]. Strategic elements of cortical circuitry are synaptic contacts: sites of neuronal interaction. If we first determine the location of early formed synapses, we may then seek the pre- and postsynaptic elements, that is, the structures which meet and interact at each synaptic junction.

The dynamic aspects of cortical development cannot be studied directly: neuronal growth cannot be observed in an intact brain. The pattern of development can be approached only by the analysis of static properties at multiple ages. We have selected the newborn dog as a starting point for these studies. Our observations have been restricted to a small portion of primary somesthetic cortex. This region was selected because, in mature cortex, its input and physiologic properties are relatively well known. It is particularly advantageous to study a primary sensory projection area because its morphologic development can be directly related to its functional development. (A related investigation of the ontogenesis of electrical activity in somesthetic cortex of the dog will be reported separately).

A selective review of the literature is necessary in order to place this work in the context of a few relevant phenomena of cortical development.

The developing neopallium consists of several layers which are parallel to the pial surface, namely the marginal layer, cortical plate, intermediate zone, and ependyma. The embryonic cortical plate is composed of densely packed cell bodies which arise from the ependymal layer. Superficial to the cortical plate is a relatively cell-poor band, the marginal layer; deep to the cortical plate is a thicker cell-poor region, the intermediate zone or rudimentary white matter. The adult cortex is formed from the cortical plate plus the marginal layer. The marginal layer is the primordium of layer I, and is unique in that it never contains a large number of neurons. The cortical plate will form the remainder of the cortex, layers II to VI. It is the growth of neuronal elements within the immature cortex that is especially relevant to this investigation.

Growth of Cortical Neurons. Current ideas of the maturation of cortical neurons are based largely on two principles which originated near the end of the 19th century. Vignal (1888) observed that cortical maturation begins deep in the cortical plate where the earliest cells to mature form a layer of large cells, which he recognized as the primordium of layer V. Subsequent maturation progresses through layers IV, III, and II successively[2]. (Layer VI was out of sequence in that it was the last to mature.) This developmental sequence was subsequently

---

1 A preliminary report was presented to the American Association of Anatomists (Cajal Club), Molliver and Van der Loos (1969).

2 In order to avoid confusion about cortical layers, we have translated the numbering systems used in the early literature into the current terminology, as used by Koelliker (1896) and Brodmann (1909).

presented by others (Cajal, 1906; Koelliker, 1896; Lorente de Nó, 1933; Stefanowska, 1898) in simplified form as a general principle: deep cells mature earlier than superficial cells.

The second principle, proposed by Cajal (1906), is that individual neurons follow a uniform pattern of dendrite growth, summarized in Fig. 1. Dendrites appear and grow in the following sequence: apical dendrite trunk (b in Fig. 1), terminal bouquet of apical dendrite (c), basal dendrites (d), and finally, collaterals from the apical dendrite trunk (e). Cajal proposed that spines were the last structural elements to appear, but he did not describe the sequence of their appearance over the dendritic surface.

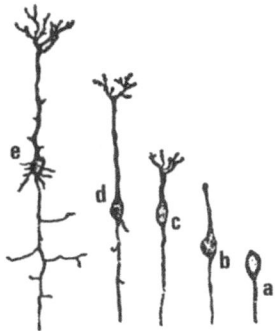

Fig. 1. Sequence (a—e) of dendrite growth proposed by Cajal. This figure taken from a drawing by Cajal (1906, 1911) illustrates that apical dendrites mature earlier than basal dendrites

In the current decade, due largely to the interest in physiologic maturation of cortex, the pattern of dendrite growth has been re-examined. Studies which we consider pertinent to the principles of Vignal and Cajal were performed in several species: mouse (Meller, Breipohl and Glees, 1968b), rat (Noback and Purpura, 1961), rabbit (Marty, 1962; Noback and Purpura, 1961), sheep (Åström, 1967), cat (Marty, 1962; Noback and Purpura, 1961), dog[3] (Fox, Inman and Himwich, 1966), and man (Conel, 1939; Rabinowicz, 1964; Schadé and Van Groenigen, 1961). Each of these investigations supported one or both of the two original principles of cortical maturation[4].

---

3 We have experienced difficulty in evaluating the description of immature dog cortex by Fox et al. (1966) due to its insufficient documentation.

4 The only stated exception to the principle that deeper cortical neurons differentiate earlier than more superficial ones is by Noback and Purpura (1961). They state that this sequence of maturation may not apply to the cat, for they observed that the basal dendrites of deep pyramids were less mature than those of more superficial pyramids in the newborn period. Their findings are in contradiction with those of Koelliker (1896), who also studied neonatal cats and confirmed the general principle that deep neurons differentiate earlier than superficial ones; he described and depicted extensively branched basal dendrites of deep large pyramidal cells (cf. his Fig. 727 and 728). In view of this discrepancy, we examined our Golgi-Cox sections from immature cats and found that basal dendrites of deep pyramids were consistently more mature than those of superficial pyramids — at birth and in fetal cats from 45 to 58 days of gestation. We are unable to explain the unique observation of Noback and Purpura.

Our acceptance of the attractive principle of Cajal (in cortical pyramidal cells, the formation of the apical dendritic bouquet precedes the growth of basal dendrites) would require that well documented, conflicting evidence be ignored. Moreover, inherent in this principle is the unwarranted assumption that all pyramids follow the same pattern of dendrite growth. In view of these considerations, our own observations have led us to question that principle.

Every relevant paper (e.g. Åström, 1967; Cajal, 1906; Lorente de Nó, 1933; Marty, 1962; Noback and Purpura, 1961; Stefanowska, 1898) confirms (with convincing documentation) that the most *superficial* pyramids have well developed apical dendrites before they have basal dendrites. However, as early as 1898, Stefanowska recognized, in newborn mice, that the large pyramids *deep* in the cortex showed the opposite pattern of growth: namely, that the numerous basal dendrites of these cells were long and sometimes branched, whereas the apical dendritic bouquet (not having yet reached layer I) was represented only by two or three short twigs (cf. p. 13—14 of her paper). Lorente de Nó (1933) appears to have recognized the same phenomenon, which is well documented in his drawings (cf. his Fig. 14 and 17). Other examples of earlier development of basal than of apical dendrites in deep neurons may be seen in the figures of Åström (1967) and Rabinowicz (1964). These observations have not previously led to any formal criticism or restatement of Cajal's principle.

We propose that Cajal's principle that apical dendrite maturation precedes that of basal dendrites is not of general validity. The available evidence indicates that cells in different layers may have different sequences of dendrite growth. In superficial pyramids, the apical dendrites develop earlier than the basal dendrites; in deep pyramids, the basal dendrites mature before the apical dendrites. By "superficial pyramids" we mean the most superficial pyramidal cells in the cortical plate; by "deep pyramids" we mean those from the deepest tier of layer III to the bottom of layer V. These two examples, superficial and deep pyramids, reveal opposite sequences of dendrite growth. The demenstration of other, possibly intermediate sequences of dendrite growth will require a quantitative analysis of Golgi material.

We shall now critically examine Vignal's principle that differentiation proceeds from deep to superficial levels of the cortex. This principle is valid for those parameters of maturation upon which it is based; it may not be valid for other parameters. That feature of cortical pyramids which most graphically conveys the impression of relative maturity is the number and extent of basal dendrites. Indeed, it is the precocity of deep basal dendrites that was the basis for proposing that deep neurons mature first (Cajal, 1906; Lorente de Nó, 1933; Vignal, 1888). Hence, the principle may be more accurately restated in a form that is in accord with the original observations of Vignal, as follows: the basal dendrites of deep pyramids mature earlier than the basal dendrites of superficial pyramids.

A notable exception to the principle that maturation proceeds from deep to superficial layers of the cortex is the maturational sequence of apical dendrite bouquets. Stefanowska (1898) showed that the apical dendrite bouquets of superficial pyramids mature earlier than those of deep pyramids[5]. This exception

_____

5 Was Lorente de Nó (1933) making this same point in his footnote on page 416 ?

may be used to emphasize that a comparison of maturity at different depths is only meaningful in respect to the parameters of development that have been compared.

The pattern of dendrite growth in immature cortex is highly relevant to this study because, in cerebral cortex, dendrites are the predominant postsynaptic elements. Those cortical loci in which there is early dendrite maturation are the most likely locations of early synapses. Lorente de Nó has described, in newborn mouse, cortical strata which contain dendritic plexuses. These strata of relatively mature dendrites correspond to pale bands in Nissl sections (Åström, 1967; Lorente de Nó, 1933). The existence of strata containing relatively mature dendrites could be a basis for predicting the early formation of synapses in those strata. However, it has not yet been shown that the spatio-temporal pattern of dendrite maturation is consistently associated with the pattern of synapse formation. That early maturing dendrites engage in synaptic contacts has been postulated on the basis of electrophysiologic observations: it was proposed that early synapses appear in relation to superficial (apical) dendrites (Bernhard, Kolmodin and Meyerson, 1967; Marty, 1962; Molliver, 1967; Purpura, Carmichael and Housepian, 1960) and also in relation to deep dendrites (Molliver, 1967).

Growth of Axons into Cortex. The growth of axons into a region of cortex from other parts of the nervous system has not been extensively investigated. Cajal reported the presence of afferent fibers in cortex of newborn rabbit (1891) and of newborn mouse (1906); these are the earliest stages that he described. Afferent fibers were observed in deep cortex of sheep early in fetal life (Åström, 1967). In newborn cats, afferent fibers were reported to reach layer IV and to form "simplified bushy arbors" (Scheibel and Scheibel, 1964); it is difficult to assess the significance of this observation, which was documented only by a schematic drawing. In maturing cortex, the study of axonal pathways is more difficult than that of dendrites due to uncertainties in the proper identification of fibers and to inconsistencies of staining.

The Retzius-Cajal Cells. A striking characteristic of immature cortex is the transient presence, in layer I, of unique cells. These are large cells which have long processes that are parallel to the pial surface. These horizontal processes emit thin ascending branches which often terminate in small subpial expansions. These cells[6] were first described by Retzius (1891, 1893) in cortex from late fetal stages of man, dog, and cat[7]: some of his original drawings are reproduced in Fig. 2. Cajal (1911) subsequently reported seeing them in perinatal mouse and man. Both Retzius and Cajal agreed that cells with the morphologic features described above could not be found after the neonatal period.

In adult cortex there are horizontal cells in layer I that are quite different from the fetal cells first described by Retzius. The adult horizontal cells lack the

---

6 Retzius (1891) first described these cells as glia but later he unequivocally identified them as neurons (1893).

7 The history of these cells is made interesting by conflicts over priority. The following statement from a recent paper (Noback and Purpura, 1961) is an example. "To our knowledge, the present and an earlier preliminary report ... provide the first description of Retzius-Cajal cells in sub-primate mammals".

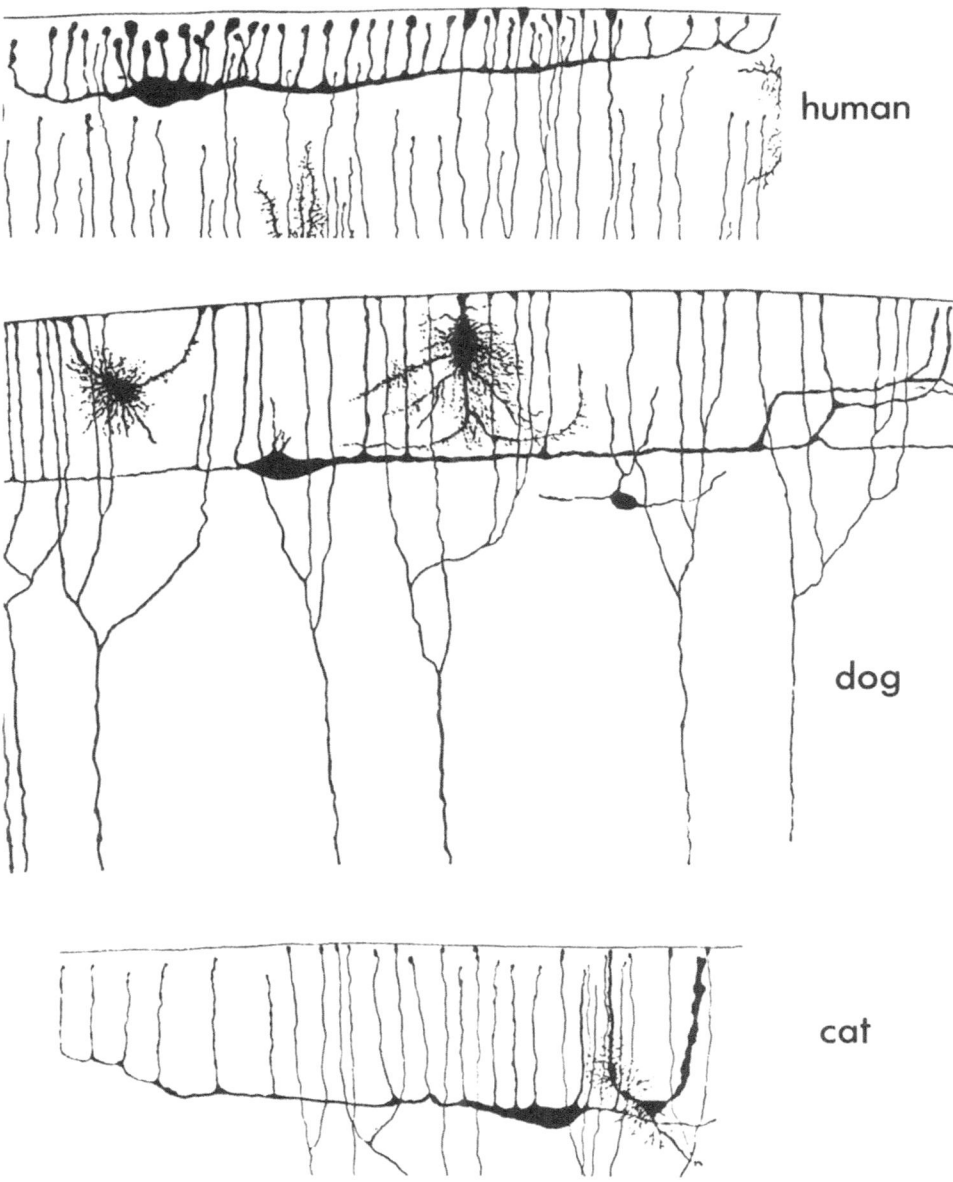

Fig. 2. Retzius-Cajal cells. These cells are taken from drawings made by Retzius (1893) (rapid Golgi method). The cells depicted here are from a seven-month human embryo, from a five-day old dog, and from a fetal cat "nearly at term"

ascending branches and are usually smaller than the fetal cells. Cajal proposed that the adult horizontal cells represent a later developmental stage of the horizontal cells found in the fetus. Due to the characteristic differences between the adult and fetal types, Cajal divided them into two morphologic classes:

"fetal form" and "adult form" of the horizontal cells. There is as yet no evidence to support Cajal's belief that these two manifestly different forms represent the same cell at different ages.

Whatever their lineage, the fetal and adult horizontal cells of layer I should be distinguished from one another. The term "Retzius-Cajal cells" (or less preferably "Cajal-Retzius cells") should be reserved for the fetal form of these cells, in accord with current terminology (Åström, 1967; Lorente de Nó, 1933; Marty, 1962; Noback and Purpura, 1961). The adult form of horizontal cell in layer I should be called "horizontal cell of Cajal", in accord with standard nomenclature (Brodal, 1969; Crosby, Humphrey and Lauer, 1962; Truex and Carpenter, 1964). We belabor the nomenclature of these cells only because misleading statements have appeared in the recent literature, due to confusion in terminology. For example, Fox and Inman (1966) failed to distinguish between the fetal and adult horizontal cells and thus concluded that typical Retzius-Cajal cells in dog cortex persist to adulthood. Meller, Breipohl and Glees (1968a) attempt to describe the maturation of horizontal cells in mouse cortex, but fail to distinguish between fetal and adult forms and even include non-horizontal cells of layer I in the same category.

Development of Cortical Synapses. The following discussion of synapse development will be restricted to papers dealing with the ultrastructure of immature neocortex. Previous electron microscopic studies of immature neocortex have revealed some properties of synapse development which are relevant to this paper. There is reported to be an early stage of cortical maturation characterized by the presence of relatively few synapses, and a subsequent stage characterized by a rapid increase in their number [in rabbit (Gruner and Zahnd, 1967), cat (Voeller, Pappas and Purpura, 1963), mouse (Meller, Breipohl and Glees, 1968b) and rat (Aghajanian and Bloom, 1967)]. The earliest synapses are axo-dendritic and are reportedly seen only on dendrites of large diameter .Axo-somatic synapses could be found only in the subsequent stage when axo-dendritic synapses had become more numerous (Meller, Breipohl and Glees, 1968b; Voeller, Pappas and Purpura, 1963).

In order to analyze the development of cortical circuitry, it is necessary to know precisely where in the cortex the earliest synapses are located. This has not been a problem of primary concern in previous electron-microscopic studies of developing neocortex.

In a study of developing rabbit cortex, Grüner and Zahnd (1967) stated that synapses were first found throughout the cortical thickness (at 20 days of gestation), later (at 10 days after birth) they were restricted to layers II-V, and subsequently (after 13 days) they were found in all layers. This unlikely sequence of synapse locations at different ages has not been confirmed.

The report by Voeller, Pappas, and Purpura (1963) of synapse development in "superficial neocortex" of kittens does not state at what depth or in which layers synapses were found, nor does it state which specific layers are encompassed by the term "superficial neocortex". The tissue examined, from fetal and neonatal kittens, was characterized as containing closely spaced cell bodies separated by groups of large dendrites. This description fits the appearance of layer II, but not that of layer I. It is not clear that layer I was included in their observations. Synapses were found almost exclusively on large dendritic trunks at that age. We cautiously interpret the results of that report as indicating that, in fetal and neonatal kittens, synapses are present on the apical dendrite trunks of pyramids with cell bodies in layer II or deeper.

In a study of developing motor cortex of mouse by Meller, Breipohl and Glees (1968b) observations were restricted specifically to layers I and II. From their report, we have with difficulty extracted the following. Synapses of layer I appear before those of layer II. Synapses in layers I and II appear on different parts of pyramidal cells in a definite sequence: first on apical dendrite shafts, then on somata and finally on basal dendrites. Although that paper also reported the later formation of several complex synaptic configurations, the description of them was obscure (cf. pp. 225—226, Meller, Breipohl and Glees, 1968b).

In a recent paper (already cited), Aghajanian and Bloom (1967) present a quantitative electron microscopic analysis of the increasing synaptic density in layer I of rat cortex during postnatal development. They use an important new method, previously introduced by them (Bloom and Aghajanian, 1966), for selective staining of synaptic membranes. If that method can be shown to reliably stain at least all synapses which can be identified with conventional methods, it will be a significant adjunct to future quantitative electron microscopic studies of synapse location during cortical maturation.

We have narrow-mindedly discussed only those problems of synapse development which are directly relevant to the analysis that we present in this report. An important phenomenon not discussed here is the changing structure of developing synapses. This problem has recently been studied and reviewed by Bunge, Bunge, and Peterson (1967).

The question to which our investigation has been directed is: *where are synapses located in immature cortex.*

The determination of synaptic location in cortex presents an interesting problem. The identification of synapses can be achieved only in the electron microscope at magnifications in the order of $10,000 \times$; it is desirable to determine the *location* of synapses in a light-microscopic image of the cortex, optimally at a magnification in the order of $100 \times$, so that cytoarchitectonic landmarks are recognizable. Therefore, it was necessary to devise a method to transpose the locations of structures identified in the electron microscope to an image of the same tissue obtained in the light microscope. Using that method in conjunction with a systematic analysis of the locations of numerous individual synapses the spatial distribution of synapses in the cerebral cortex was examined.

In this paper we shall present a quantitative method which was used to analyze the spatial distribution of synapses in the cerebral cortex. Then data will be presented from the study of primary somesthetic cortex of dog at a single stage of development: the newborn period. Finally, we shall discuss the possible relevance of these data to the development of cortical circuitry and to electrophysiologic properties of immature cortex.

Methods

Specimen Preparation

Animals. Electron microscopic (EM) data derived from three neonatal dogs are presented in this paper. The animals were bred and whelped under uniform conditions in our breeding colony. The dogs used in this study were sacrificed on the day of birth, approximately 12 hours after delivery. (The normal canine gestation is 63 days.) The three dogs, designated I, II, and III, are beagles, each of different lineage.

Dog I was born of a phenotypic beagle, laboratory reference No. D 12; tissue block *b* analyzed. Dog II was a purebred beagle, laboratory reference No. B 3; block *b* analyzed. Dog III was also a purebread beagle, laboratory reference No. B 10; block *a* analyzed. The weight of each dog was as follows: I 266 g, II 240 g, III 330 g.

Tissue Removal. Following careful craniotomy, small blocks of cortex were removed with a razor blade fragment. The blocks of cortex measured $1 \times 1 \times 2$ mm and were taken from somesthetic cortex (S I). The lateral portion of post-cruciate gyrus was used in this study, specifically the area of representation of the contralateral forelimb digits (Hamuy, Bromiley and Woolsey, 1956). The analyzed block from Dog I was taken from the anterior portion of this area; analyzed blocks from Dogs II and III were from mid portion, i.e., crest of gyrus.

Fixation. Initial fixation was obtained with 2.5 % glutaraldehyde in sodium phosphate buffer (formula: sodium monophosphate 33.8 g + sodium di-phosphate 3.3 g + 50 % glutaraldehyde 50 cc + H_2O 960 cc). The buffer osmolarity was 320 mOsm prior to the addition of glutaraldehyde; pH was maintained at 7.4. Tissue from Dogs I and II was fixed by immersion of the blocks in buffered glutaraldehyde for three hours at $4°$ C. Animal III was perfused with the same fixative; a volume of 250 cc was injected into the aortic arch through a catheter inserted via the abdominal aorta. Cortical blocks from this animal were placed in buffered glutaraldehyde for three hours.

Following fixation, all blocks were washed several times in the same buffer and then placed in 1 % osmium tetroxide (same buffer) for three hours at $4°$ C. The blocks were again washed in the buffer and then dehydrated in a graded ethanol series.

Embedding. In anticipation of the special handling of blocks in this study it was necessary to use a soft embedding medium that can easily be trimmed without chipping, and which consistently yields adjacent thick and thin sections. The following mixture of epoxy resins satisfies these requirements and was used (modified from a formula suggested by LKB Instruments, Inc.):

Araldite 502 (Durcupan A/M)	20 parts
Epon 812	25 parts
DDSA	60 parts
DMP-30	1.5 parts

Propylene oxide was used as the intermediary between alcohol and epoxy resin. The embedding sequence of Luft (1961) was followed. The blocks were placed in the final epoxy batch in flat silicone rubber molds and cured as follows: $35°$ C 12 hours, $45°$ C 8 hours, $60°$ C 12 hours (or more). (We observed that the duration of cure at $45°$ C is a major determinant of ultimate hardness. *Longer* times at $45°$ C yield a *softer* block after complete cure.)

Specimen Preparation, General. Sections were cut on a Reichert Om U2 ultra-microtome, especially advantageous because sectioning can be interrupted and resumed without resetting the distance between specimen and knife. Glass knives made with an LKB Knifemaker were used. Thin sections are mounted on a formvar film. In the mounting procedure, water trapped between the section and the formvar evaporates leaving a residue under the section. For this reason, extreme precautions must be taken to maintain cleanliness. We have found it desirable to use triple-distilled water in the knife trough and in all subsequent steps in which sections are placed in water. This water has a substantially lower sediment upon evaporation than has single- or double-distilled water. Reagent grade acetone has much sediment and it may not be used. It was noted that triple-distilled water has unusually favorable physical properties in the knife trough (e.g. non-wetting of knife face, good section flotation, easy separation and pick-up of sections).

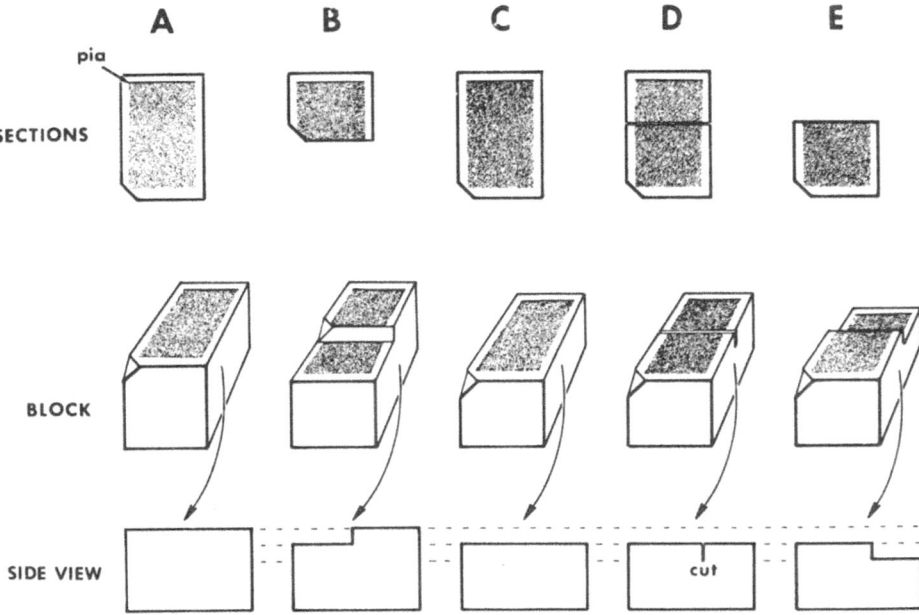

Fig. 3. Block trimming. Method used to obtain sections of superficial and deep cortex for electron microscopy. *Sections A, B, C, etc.*, are cut from upper surfaces of *Blocks A, B, C, etc. Side views* of block appear in bottom row. Operations described in text

Sections used for this study had interference colors ranging from pale gold to pale silver. After being mounted on formvar, the sections were stained with uranyl acetate and lead citrate (Venable and Coggeshall, 1965) and then carbon coated. Thick sections were cut at 1—2 μ thickness and mounted unstained for examination by phase contrast microscopy. Harleco synthetic resin (dissolved in toluene) is used as the mounting medium since it gives the best phase contrast image and the least wrinkling of all resins tried by us. It is difficult to obtain aesthetically satisfying low-power phase contrast photomicrographs[8]. This drawback was accepted in order to eliminate the possibility of damaging critical thick sections during a staining procedure.

Special methods for block trimming and section mounting will now be described in detail.

Block Trimming. In order to study the distribution of synapses throughout the cortical depth, it would be desirable to obtain thin sections that include the entire cortical thickness. However, the cortex usually exceeds 1 mm in thickness, and thin sections are preferably limited in size to less than 1 mm on any side. Thus, in order to examine the entire cortical depth it was necessary to obtain two overlapping series of sections from deep and superficial regions of the cortex. It is essential subsequently to reconstruct the cortex so that the depths of all structures within it may be known relative to the pia mater. Therefore, the deep and superficial sections should be from parallel planes as close together as possible. We have attempted to resolve these problems in the following way, as illustrated in Fig. 3.

A block of tissue embedded in epoxy is oriented in the microtome so that thick sections ($>1\,\mu$) through the entire cortex are cut perpendicular to the pial surface

---

8 It was not possible, using the Leitz (Zernike) phase-contrast system, to obtain evenly illuminated photomicrographs. Moderately acceptable micrographs were made only after substantial (improvised) modification of the equipment. (Details available on request.)

(Fig. 3A). These sections are inspected with phase contrast to judge whether the plane of sectioning is parallel to the predominant orientation of cells and cell streams; corrections are made by angular adjustments of the block axis. The block is then trimmed so that a sliver parallel to the block face is removed from the deep part of the cortex; the sliver is about 0.1—0.2 mm thick (Fig. 3B). Several thick sections are then cut and mounted on slides, and adjacent thin sections are cut and mounted on grids. These sections contain superficial cortex and include the pial surface. After approximately ten thin sections have been retrieved, thick sections are cut repeatedly until a section passes through the entire block face. This last section is saved (Fig. 3C) and is later used for the spatial representation of our data. A shallow cut (0.2 mm deep) is made into the block face, perpendicular to the plane of section (Fig. 3D) and about 1 mm above the deep edge of the cortex. Then a few thick sections are cut. Two sections come off with each pass of the knife and these are saved in pairs (Fig. 3D). They are later to be superimposed on the section which goes through the entire block face (Fig. 3 C), and the cut edge is used to determine the location of the ad-pial border of the deep section. The portion of the block face containing superficial cortex is then removed by undercutting (Fig. 3E), and several thick sections (of deep cortex) are cut and saved. Then a series of approximately ten thin sections is cut and mounted on grids. These sections containing deep cortex are adjacent to thick section E. Note that the cut in step D is made such that the superficial and deep sections overlap. A corner is always cut off so that the orientation of sections can be easily maintained in subsequent procedures.

Synapses observed in both superficial and deep thin sections are located by reference to adjacent thick sections 3B and 3E, respectively. The synaptic locations in these sections are, in turn, transposed to section 3C in order to combine both sets of data (i.e., deep and superficial) on a single scale of cortical depth. Examples of this method will be shown below. (Note that the full thickness sections shown in Figs. 17—19 correspond to section C in Fig. 3).

Mounting of Thin Sections. Thin sections for EM examination are mounted on single hole grids covered with a formvar film. Our adoption of this (tedious) method is based on the following considerations. The analysis of a tissue, such as cortex, which has a distinct geometric organization is facilitated by having the entire section available for inspection, unobstructed by grid bars. Our sampling method, described below, requires an unobstructed field. The determination of section orientation and the identification of large structures, e.g., cell bodies and pial surface, are facilitated by the use of single-hole grids.

Copper grids with a single round hole, 1 mm in diameter, are preferred. Grids with an oval 1 × 3 mm hole were tried and rejected because they had a high incidence of rupture of the sections (due to uneven stress on the film because of the unequal axes of the hole).

The thin sections were mounted according to a method derived from Gay and Anderson (1954). A formvar film was cast upon water and picked up on wire loops 5 mm in diameter. Sections cut on triple-distilled water are transferred, using a platinum loop, to a beaker of water. Under a dissecting microscope the section is picked up on a formvar covered loop and dried. This loop carrying the section on a formvar film is then inspected by means of interference colors (under a stereo-microscope with vertical illumination). A copper grid is cleaned and a small piece is cut from its edge to provide an orientation mark. The grid is dipped into 1% polybutane in xylene (3-M Company) to improve its adherence to the formvar film. After drying, the grid is picked up by vacuum applied through a length of steel hypodermic tubing held in a micro-manipulator (Leitz). Under microscopic observation and using the manipulator controls, the grid is oriented such that the section is centered in the grid hole and the pial edge is parallel to the cut edge of the grid. The grid is then dropped over the section by interruption of the vacuum. The grid is gently pressed down, and the formvar is trimmed away using the sharp point of a disposable hypodermic needle. Finally, the grid is lifted free with forceps. Slight heating of the air (to about 45° C) during this process decreases the fragility of the formvar. *Gentle* treatment of the grid with a stream of ozone (Kodak static eliminating device) improves adherence of the formvar and eliminates the catastrophes caused by static electrical charges on the grid.

The specimens are then stained by floating, section side down, on a drop of stain. The grids are dried by inserting each one into a short length of 3 mm i.d. plastic tubing mounted on a rod. (If grids are placed on a flat surface when wet, the film will sag, contact the surfacs,

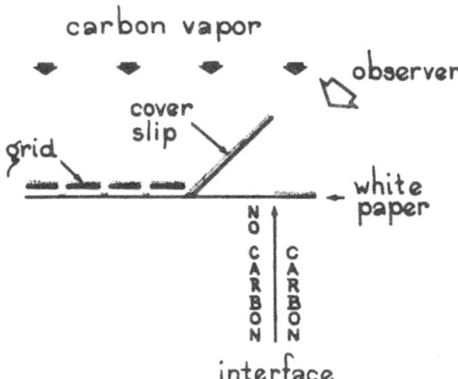

Fig. 4. Technique for judging thickness of carbon film during evaporation procedure (side view represented). Cover slip shields portion of paper from carbon, thereby producing an interface which is visible through the glass wall of the vacuum chamber

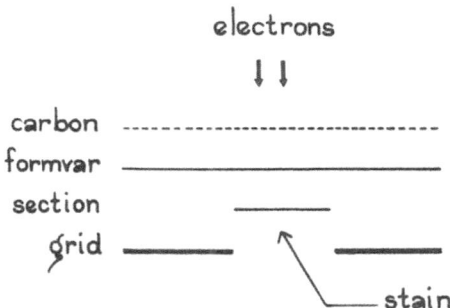

Fig. 5. Schematic cross-sectional view of complete specimen, as mounted in electron microscope

and break). The grids are then placed in a Balzer BA-3 vacuum evaporator and a thin film of carbon is evaporated on the formvar surface to improve its thermal stability. The thickness of the carbon film is judged by placing a tilted cover slip at 45° to a white paper in the path of the carbon vapor (Fig. 4). A shadow is cast on the paper producing an interface which can be observed from outside the vacuum chamber. A pale tan colored film of carbon is adequate for stabilization. The specimens are inspected for gross defects in an incident light microscope. They are then ready for examination in the electron microscope.

Fig. 5 summarizes the position of each layer in the final specimen. The grid is placed in the electron beam so that the section faces the fluorescent screen and the carbon faces the electron source. Using the cut edge of the grid as an orienting marker, the specimen is mounted in the electron microscope such that the pial surface is parallel to one axis of the stage movement.

Golgi Methods. Blocks of somesthetic cortex from beagles on the day of birth (littermates of dogs used for EM study) were fixed and impregnated by a Golgi-Cox method (Van der Loos, 1959). Celloidin embedded blocks were sectioned at 100 μ for light microscopic study. Some sections were treated (destained) to partially remove the Cox impregnation in order to render the cells semi-translucent (Van der Loos, in prep.) This method is of particular value in immature cortex in which neurons tend to be impregnated in clusters, obscuring their individual characteristics. Additional sections of 30 μ thickness were stained by a Nissl method (methylene blue-Cl) after the Cox impregnation was completely removed.

The presentation of Golgi-Cox data demonstrates our approach to the problem of relating synaptic locations and post-synaptic elements in immature cortex. The cells presented are those we subjectively deem typical of our material; they are not the result of a systematic analysis of cell types in immature cortex.

Data Collection

The thin sections are examined systematically in a Philips EM-200 electron microscope in order to determine the distribution of synapses in cortical depth. Of each section inspected in the electron microscope, a narrow strip of tissue (ca. $6\,\mu \times 800\,\mu$), approximately perpendicular to the pia, is examined in its entirety and recorded on film via a series of overlapping micrographs. Every suspicious synapse is noted, and its location within the section recorded. Synapses are located with respect to cortical cytoarchitectonics by transposing each synaptic location to the light micrograph of an adjacent thick section. The steps in this analysis will now be described in detail.

The analysis of a strip of tissue is called a "probe". The entire specimen is moved through the electron beam in a straight line approximately perpendicular to the pial surface. The linear movement is obtained by turning only one stage micrometer, the scale of which is calibrated in $1\,\mu$ divisions. Displacement of the specimen is read directly from the micrometer scale and is recorded for every photograph. (The accuracy of reading the displacement is $\pm 0.5\,\mu$; accuracy of replacing the specimen after its removal from the column is $\pm 1\,\mu$).

Two methods of performing a probe were used in this study. Our initial probes were selectively photographed. The tissue to be analyzed was carefully inspected in the electron microscope using the binocular microscope and a fine grain fluorescent screen. When any apposition was deemed a "suspicious synapse", a photograph was taken. Areas not containing possible synapses were not photographed. The width of strip analyzed ($2.5\,\mu$) was determined by the field of view of the binocular microscope.

A more efficient method of probe selection was later developed. In this second method, the strip of tissue ($6\,\mu$ wide) to be analyzed was photographed in its entirety by taking successive overlapping electron micrographs at intervals of $5\,\mu$. Tissue was not analyzed in the electron microscope, and only sufficient time was taken to focus, so that contamination was minimized. By subsequent examination of the films, the entire strip of tissue could be analyzed at leisure by both investigators. The area of tissue inspected per probe was greater with this method because the width of the inspected strip was much greater.

Over 2,000 electron micrographs were taken on 35 mm film, Eastman Fine Grain Release Positive. The most useful film magnification was found to be $4,875 \times$. Films were inspected at $10 \times$. For final inspection selected exposures were printed at a total magnification of $33,000 \times$.

A method was developed to accurately locate all points along a probe with reference to the cytoarchitectonic pattern of the cortex. Use was made of our observation that the area of the specimen examined in the electron microscope is clearly marked by the electron beam. When a specimen is exposed to the beam, changes in its electron opacity occur as a function of time. These changes occur in two stages. During the first stage (duration about 100 sec in our material) there is an increased electron lucency of the specimen, manifested by a brighter image on the screen and an increased image contrast. Continued exposure to the electron beam produces the second stage: decreased electron lucency and loss of image contrast, a phenomenon often referred to as contamination. These changes are sharply restricted to the area of the section exposed to the electron beam. When using the double condenser system, a narrow beam ($10—25\,\mu$ diameter) may be obtained, and the location of the inspected area can be accurately defined.

When a probe has been completed, the entire section is photographed in the electron microscope at a magnification of approximately $30 \times$. Under these conditions, the inspected area is seen as an electron-lucent band (cf. Fig. 7).

An alternative method exists for visualizing the location of the inspected area of the section. With an incident light microscope (e.g. Leitz Ortholux with "Opak" illuminator) interference colors can be obtained which reveal the tissue and the inspected area in brilliant contrasting colors (see Fig. 6).

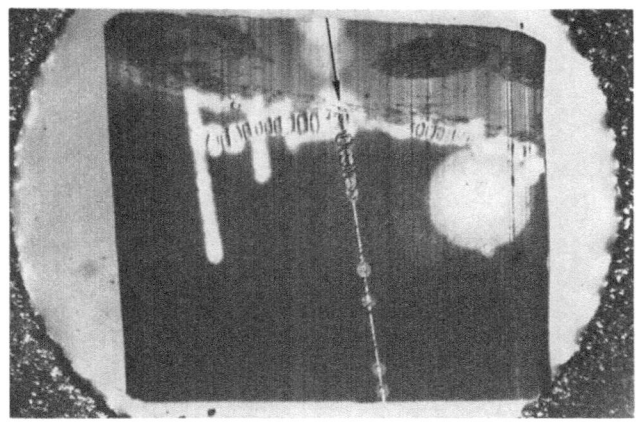

Fig. 6. Incident-light photomicrograph of thin section after inspection in electron microscope. Arrow points to probe. Pale areas result from brief exposure to electron beam. Dark core within pale area indicates contamination produced by prolonged exposure to electron beam. Pale areas other than probe betray preliminary inspection of the tissue. In reality, pale and dark areas are represented by brilliant, contrasting interference colors (e.g., gold and blue). Circular border is grid. Hole diameter 1 mm

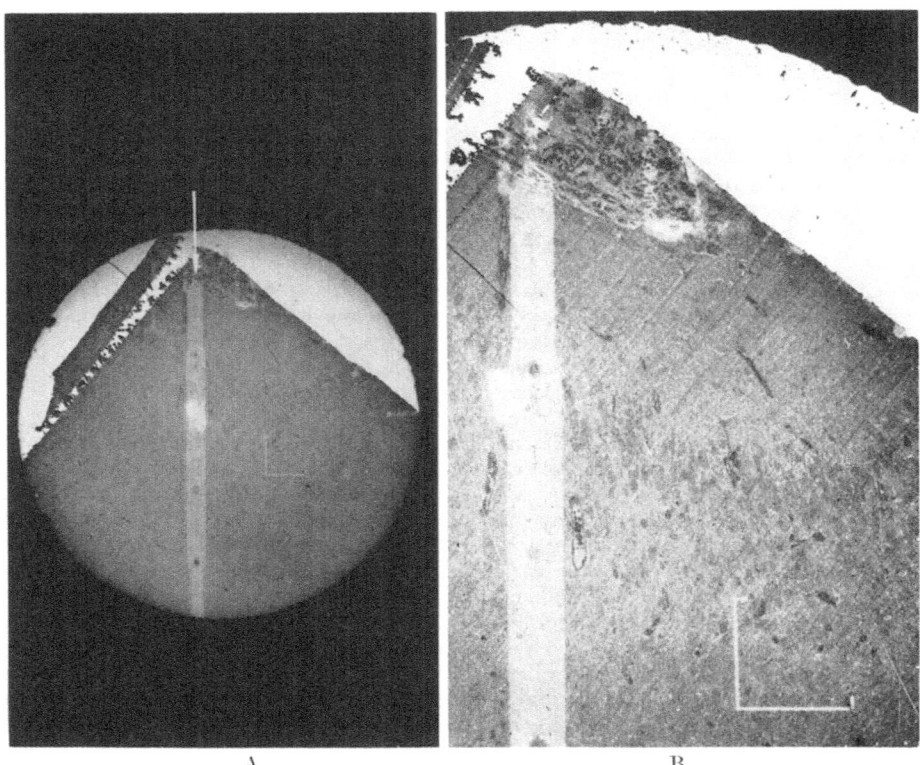

A   B

Fig. 7. "Electron marking" of section—the procedure used to show probe location (Probe 7, Dog I). *A:* Low power electron micrograph of thin section. The pale, electron lucent band (at arrow) indicates the location of probe. The circular field of view is produced by the grid hole. Right angle magnification scale is engraved by electron beam; each arm = 100 μ.
B: Detail of *A.* Note resolution of structural details, which can also be found in light micrograph of adjacent thick section (Fig. 8 B)

2*

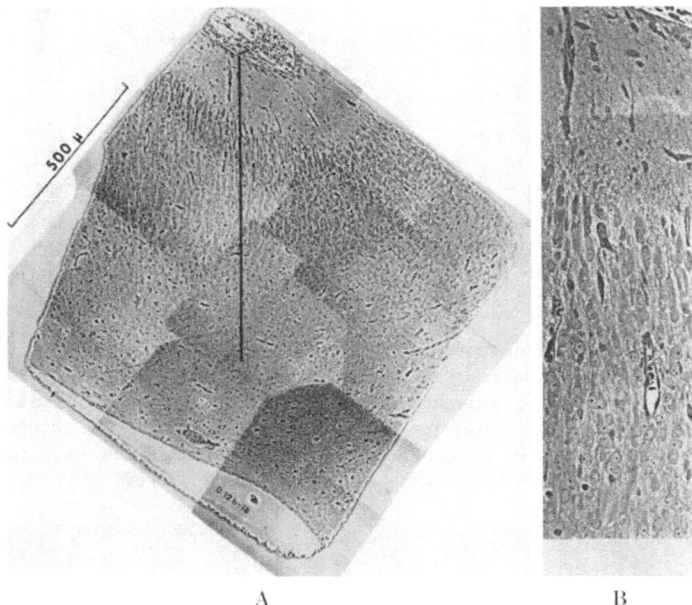

A   B

Fig. 8. Phase contrast photomicrographs of thick section adjacent to thin section shown in Fig. 7. To facilitate comparison, Figs. 7 and 8 have same orientation. *A:* The black line in this collage indicates the location of the probe seen in the electron micrograph (Fig. 7). *B:* Detail of *A* taken from region of probe; note pia in upper part of picture. Relate to Fig. 7B

A magnification scale can be placed directly on the section by virtue of the same phenomenon. With the 2nd condenser focussed to cross-over, the specimen is displaced by a known distance (e.g. 100 μ) along each axis of stage movement. This procedure leaves a permanent electron-lucent right-angled marker on the specimen. The length of each arm of the marker is equal to the corresponding stage displacement (in this case 100 μ).

Figure 7A is the low-power electron micrograph of a complete section revealing the location of a probe (Dog I, Probe 7). An enlarged area of this micrograph (Fig. 7B) reveals that major tissue landmarks are resolvable (e.g., blood vessels, pia, cut tissue borders, large cell bodies). These same structures can also be recognized in the adjacent thick section (Fig. 8B) and are used to accurately superimpose the low power electron micrograph upon the light micrograph of the adjacent thick section at the same magnification. This super-imposition is carried out by optically projecting the electron micrograph upon a photo-micrograph of the thick section. The location of the probe can then be precisely transposed onto the thick section photograph (cf. Fig. 8A).

The transposition process serves several functions in this study: all micrographs in a probe may be located with respect to cytoarchitectonics; the coordinates of all points along a probe may be converted to values of true sub-pial depth; data from multiple probes can then be combined; data from different animals also may be compared by using cytoarchitectonic landmarks. An additional feature of this method is that a cell examined in the electron microscope can be precisely located and identified in a photomicrograph of an adjacent thick section.

Data Analysis

In this section, the methods used for analyzing the spatial distribution of synapses will be described. All synapses were placed into classes defined by depth under the pia. The frequency distribution of synapses per depth-class

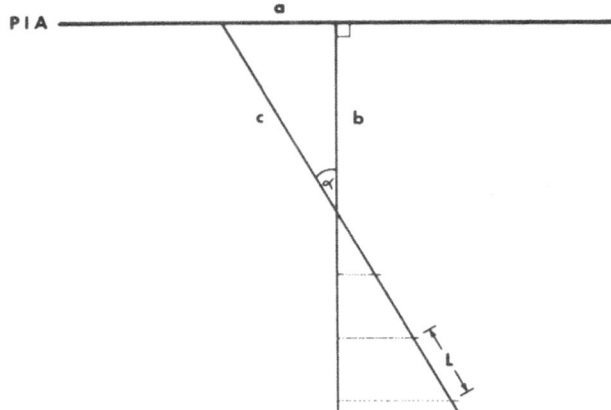

Fig. 9. Conversion of probe depth to cortical depth. Purpose: to divide probe into segments which traverse 50 μ of cortical depth. Symbols: *abc* is a right triangle; *c* is portion of probe; *b* is portion of local radial axis; α is angle between probe and local radial axis. Method: Determine length (*L*) of probe segment which projects upon a 50 μ segment of the local radial axis. COSα = b/c; hence, when b = 50 μ, L = 50/COSα. Then, beginning at pia, divide probe into successive segments of length *L*

was then determined. The problem of defining a synapse was approached by placing each suspicious interneuronal apposition into one of several morphologically distinct groups. The steps in this analysis will now be described in detail.

Determination of Depth-Classes. The depth of each synapse must be known with reference to the pia. The term "cortical depth" is here defined as the distance between the pia and a sub-pial point along a line parallel to the cortical cell streams. This line, which we call the *local radial axis*, is often approximately perpendicular to the pia. Due to the irregular curvature of the cortex, the local radial axis changes from one region to another; it is therefore determined for each probe.

The probes are not precisely parallel to the local radial axis but — due to uncertainties in section orientation — at a small angle to them. Thus, the "depth" of a point along a probe is not equal to the "cortical depth" of that point. The positions of all points in a probe must be converted to values in the scale of cortical depth.

The conversion of probe depth to cortical depth is performed in the following manner. A line representing the local radial axis is drawn through the midpoint of each probe. Since the probe data will be placed in 50 μ depth classes, a distance (L) along the probe which projects onto a 50 μ segment of the radial axis must be determined (see Fig. 9). Beginning at the pia, the probe is divided into segments of length L. The cortical depth of each segment is now given by its projection on the radial axis. All synapses within each segment of the probe are placed in the corresponding 50 μ depth-class.

In addition to placing all synapses into depth-classes, the inspected area of tissue per depth-class was calculated. This is determined differently for the two kinds of probes that were performed.

STRUCTURE   IMAGE

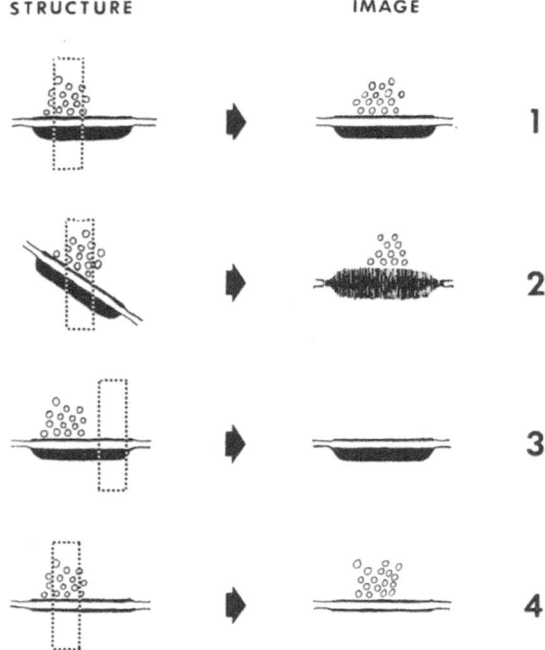

Fig. 10. Synaptic grades 1—4: morphologic features (images) and the postulated structures from which they arise. Each dotted rectangle represents the side view of a section through a synapse. Arrows indicate the direction of the electron beam as it passes through the sections to produce the images shown. The diagnostic features used to classify definite synapses are shown schematically

For the selectively photographed probes, the total area of each probe was obtained by multiplying the length of the probe by its width. (Probe length equals the total displacement of the section in the electron microscope, as read from the stage micrometer. Probe width is found by dividing the diameter of the inspected image by the image magnification.) The total probe area divided by the number of depth-classes in that probe yields the area of inspected tissue per class.

Those probes photographed in their entirety are composed of partially overlapping squares, i.e., the photographs. The non-over-lapping area of tissue in each photograph is multiplied by the number of photographs in each depth-class. The product obtained represents the total area of tissue which contributed its synapses to each depth-class in that probe.

Data from multiple probes in one animal are combined by adding the numbers of synapses in equivalent depth-classes. In order to make all depth-classes comparable, the results are expressed as the number of synapses per 1,000 square micra of inspected tissue in each depth-class. (The actual number of synapses is multiplied by an "area factor" which equals $1,000 \div$ area (in μ^2) inspected in each class. The area factors used are included in Table 1. In this

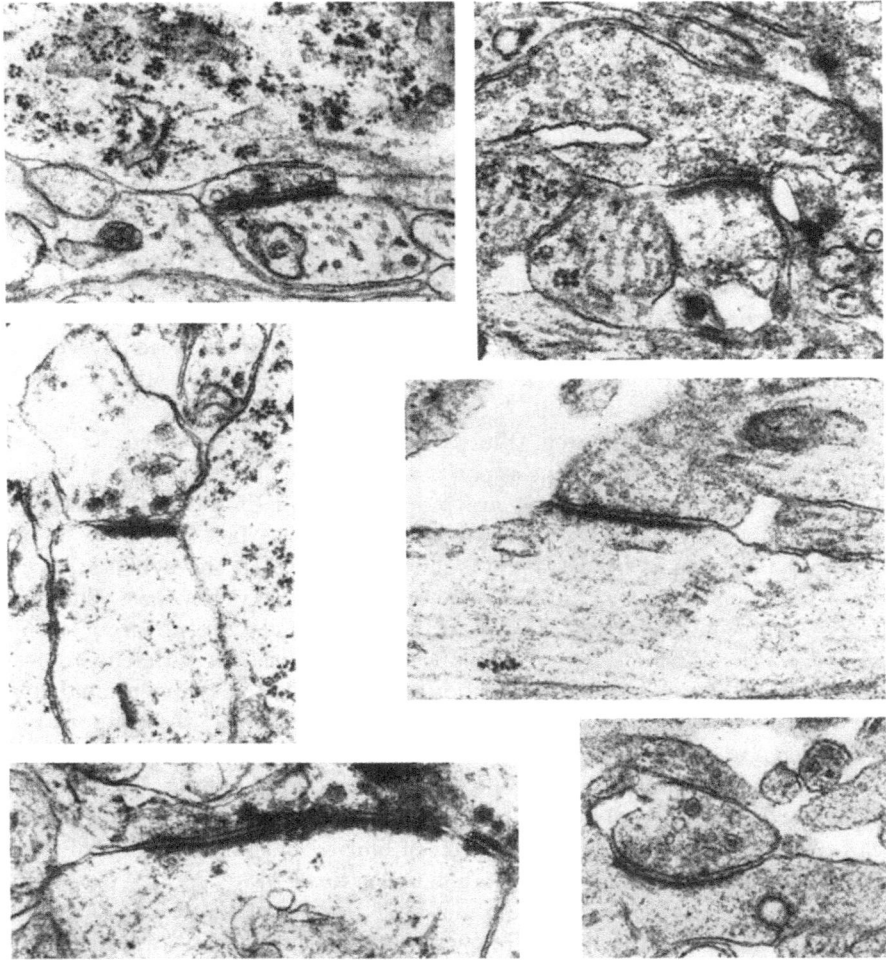

Fig. 11. Synapses of grade 1. For criteria see text. In three of the examples shown, the presynaptic elements contain some dark-core vesicles. All synapses shown in this and subsequent figures are part of the data used in this investigation. Magn. ×30,000

manner, data from equivalent depth-classes in multiple probes are combined and then corrected so that each depth-class represents an equal inspected area.)

Classification of Synapses. In qualitative electron microscopic studies it is deemed sufficient to select "typical" examples of synapses to demonstrate their morphologic features. Unusual or equivocal interneuronal appositions may be safely disregarded. In a quantitative analysis of synaptic distributions it is necessary to confront *every* suspicious apposition and to classify it. This problem is especially relevant in immature cortex where there is substantial uncertainty in the morphologic diagnosis of a synapse. In order to consistently answer the question, "What is a synapse?", we have classified all suspicious appositions into six grades based on objective morphologic criteria. We have used this classification not to analyze synaptic morphology, but only to objectify the diagnosis of synapse vs. non-synapse.

Features of synaptic grades 1 to 4 are diagrammed in Fig. 10. Examples of each grade are presented in Figs. 11—13. The structural features which determine the grading of each synapse will be noted below.

Grade 1: Cleft and both membranes are visible. Asymmetric membrane specialization. Vesicles in pre-synaptic element.

Grade 2: Cleft is obscured. Blurred membrane specialization. Vesicles in presynaptic element.

Grade 3: Cleft and both membranes are visible. Definite asymmetric membrane specialization. No vesicles.

Grade 4: Cleft is characterized by uniform membrane spacing and often contains interlemmal elements. Both membranes are specialized and symmetrical. Vesicles in presynaptic element.

Grade 5: Cleft is obscured. Blurred membrane specialization. No vesicles.

Grade 6: All other suspicious appositions.

Appositions of grades 1 to 4 are judged to be definite synapses and have been used for data analysis. In order to exclude false positives from our final results, appositions of grades 5 and 6 are *not* included in the synaptic distributions. In doing this, a small number of synapses may have been discarded.

Synaptic configurations of grades 1, 2 and 3 may result from identical three-dimensional structures which have been sectioned at different angles, as shown in Fig. 10. A grade 1 apposition is the profile (two-dimensional image) of a synapse with asymmetrical membrane specializations; the synapse is sectioned perpendicular to the apposed membranes. The most asymmetric synapses of this group are similar to Gray's (1959) type I. In an oblique section through the synapse, the pre- and postsynaptic membranes would overlap in the electron beam; the resulting image would be that of blurred membranes with obliteration of the cleft as is characteristic of grade 2 appositions.

Grade 3 synapses may contain no vesicles. Alternatively, the absence of vesicles in grade 3 may result from the section simply not including vesicles which are present; this is likely in young cortex because immature synapses contain fewer vesicles than do mature synapses, and the vesicles are often grouped in small clusters. Appositions of grade 4 represent a different 3-dimensional structure characterized by symmetrical membranes and the presence of vesicles, similar to Gray's type II. The membrane specialization (in grade 4) is less prominent than in appositions exhibiting membrane asymmetry. Thus, grade 4 appositions sectioned obliquely would probably not be recognized as specialized. Many synaptic clefts contain numerous dark lines perpendicular to the synaptolemma. These interlemmal elements (Van der Loos, 1963) are seen most often in grade 4 appositions.

Grade 5 appositions (Fig. 13A and B) have two elements of uncertainty: blurred membranes and no vesicles. Thus, they are excluded from our synapse distributions. Grade 6 appositions constitute a heterogeneous and even more uncertain group (see Fig. 13C—E). Its contents include: symmetrical membrane specializations without vesicles, profiles containing vesicles without definite associated membrane specializations and elements suggestive of synapses but with

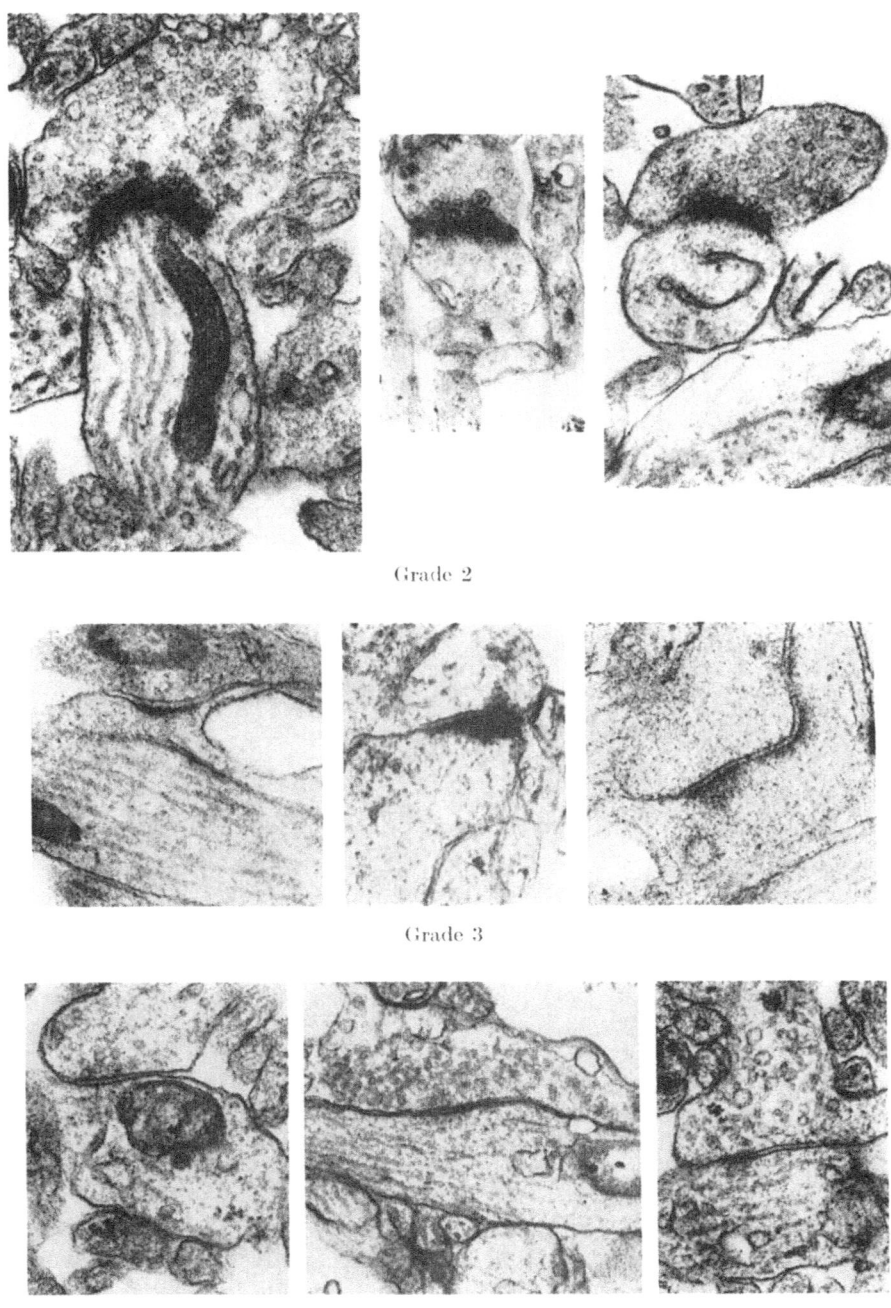

Grade 2

Grade 3

Grade 4

Fig. 12. Examples of synapses of grades 2, 3 and 4. For criteria see text and Fig. 10.
Magn. ×28,500 (grade 2); magn. ×30,000 (grade 3); magn. ×27,000 (grade 4)

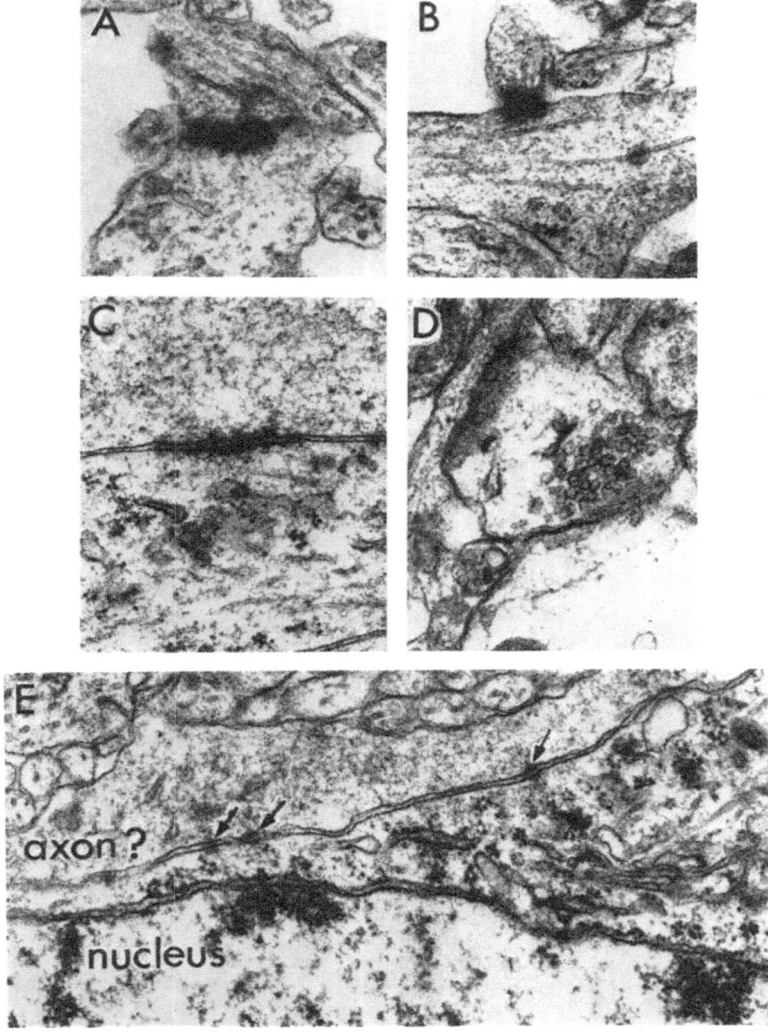

Fig. 13. Suspicious interneuronal appositions. For criteria see text. *A*, *B:* grade 5; *C*, *D*, *E:*
grade 6. Examples of grade 6 include symmetrical membrane specialization without vesicles (*C*),
profile with vesicles but no definite membrane specialization (*D*), and suspicious (at arrows)
axo-somatic apposition (*E*) (identification of axon is uncertain). Magn. ×30,000

poor definition of their morphologic features. Grade 6 consists of elements
that would usually be discarded in a qualitative study of synapses. We have
retained them, in a separate grade, in order to minimize the risk of discard-
ing synapses that have not yet developed mature properties. In immature
cortex, we are dealing with a population in flux and we do not know *a priori*
what a synapse is. The value of preserving such a group lies in forming a
collection of uncertain appositions which we can study for the emergence of
recurrent configurations.

The relative proportions of all six synaptic grades were compared for different depths and different animals. The distribution in depth of grades 5 and 6 closely matched the distribution of grade 1 to 4 appositions. Thus, there is no reason to assume that grades 5 and 6 represent a distinct population of synapses; their exclusion does not alter the form of the synaptic distributions.

In the synaptic distributions to be presented, all synapses in grades 1 to 4 from one animal are combined and treated as a single group. The synapses in grades 1 to 4 represent 75% of the total number of appositions; grades 5 to 6 include 25%. Combining the data from the three animals presented, the relative proportions of synapses in each grade from 1 to 4 is as follows:

Grade	%
1	28
2	30
3	28
4	14
Total	100% ($n = 697$)

These proportions suggest that asymmetric synapses are approximately 7 times more common than symmetric ones (in the tissue examined), assuming that grades 1 to 3 represent asymmetric synapses.

Results

The distribution of synaptic contacts for each animal will be presented in relation to the laminar cytoarchitectonic pattern of the cortex. By using cytoarchitectonic landmarks, synaptic distributions from different animals and different ages may be meaningfully compared. The determination of synaptic locations (in relation to perikaryal layers) is also used to delineate loci in which we may identify the postsynaptic elements. The cytoarchitectonic features of newborn somesthetic cortex will be described, and then the distributions of synaptic contacts will be presented.

Cytoarchitectonic Pattern. The primary somesthetic cortex of a newborn dog is shown in a low-power photomicrograph of a section through the entire hemisphere wall (Fig. 14). The ependymal layer remains prominent at this age, and cells appear to be migrating through the intermediate zone. The cortex is approximately 1 mm thick and presents two outstanding architectural features. (1) The molecular layer is thick, pale and cell-poor; it is sharply demarcated from the subjacent cortex, which has a very high cell density. (2) Near the center of the cortex is a prominent layer composed primarily of large cells. The other layers of newborn cortex are not easily delineated. Therefore, the characteristic 6-layered pattern of adult granular cortex is not apparent in the newborn dog.

That the neonatal cortex is in a stage of active neuronal growth is suggested by the presence of numerous so-called "growth cones" seen with the electron microscope (Fig. 15).

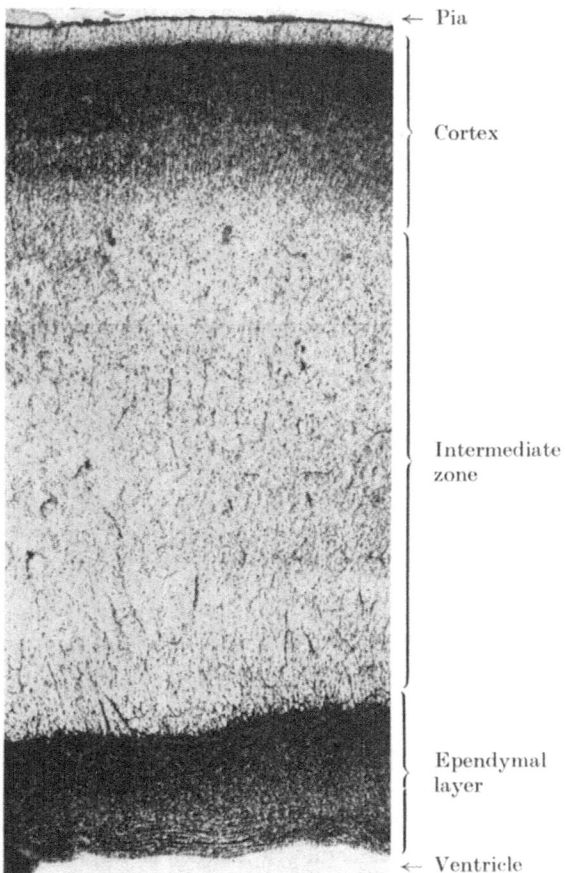

← Pia

Cortex

Intermediate
zone

Ependymal
layer

← Ventricle

Fig. 14. Cross-section through hemisphere wall—postcruciate gyrus of dog at birth. Nissl
method (Golgi-Cox, destained, methylene blue-Cl). Magn. ×25

We have attempted to identify the cytoarchitectonic layers of neonatal cortex
with respect to corresponding layers of mature cortex. The method used was
to follow the development of the outstanding cell layers of postcruciate gyrus
in brains taken from a closely spaced ontogenetic series. We have examined
Nissl-stained cortex from dogs of 0, 5, 10, 12, 18 and 30 days of age. By
30 days of age, the cytoarchitectonic pattern of the cortex is essentially mature.

The two outstanding cell layers of neonatal cortex were readily traced through
our entire series of brains. The pale molecular layer of newborn cortex will
clearly become layer I of mature cortex. The easily recognized layer of large
cells (cf. Fig. 22) deep in newborn cortex is the primordium of layer V in the
adult. This layer of large cells is shown at 5, 12, and 30 days in Fig. 16.
The cortex of the 5 day dog is very similar to that of the 0 day dog. From
0 to 5 days, layer IV is not a clearly separate entity, but it may later
be derived from the small neurons which lie above the large cell layer and

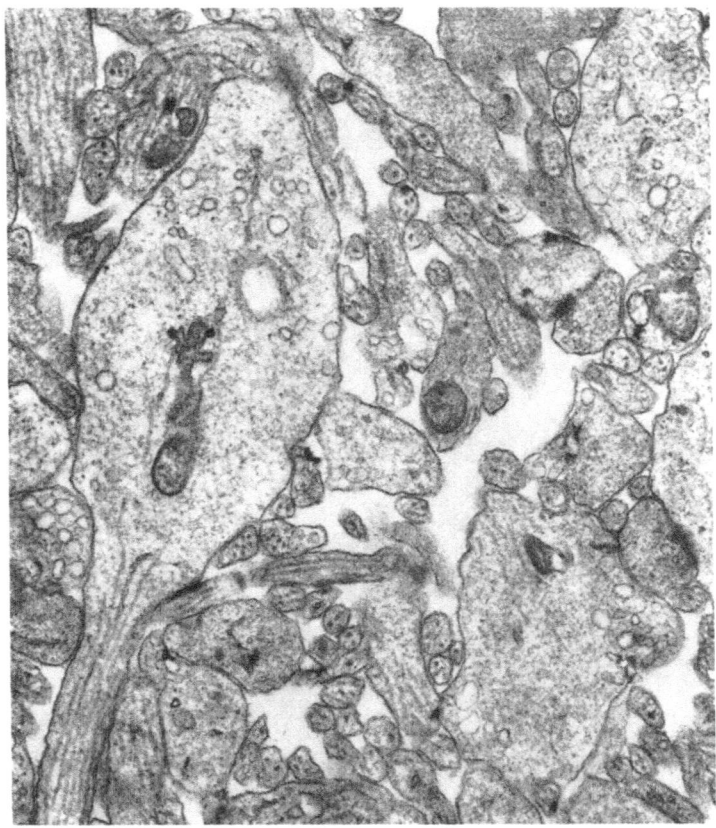

Fig. 15. Dog cortex at birth: growth cone. Is this the sign of a growing neuronal process?
Note two synapses on the right side. Electron micrograph at ×19,500

from some that are intermingled with the large cells. Such relationships between cell layers at different ages may be proposed only tenuously, because the
layers and their constituent cells may move or be transformed during ontogenesis.

Distributions of Synaptic Contacts in Three Neonatal Dogs. The locations of
all probes, from which synaptic data have been derived, are shown on photographs of thick sections which pass through the entire cortex (Figs. 17—19).
Each of these sections has been cut from the block used for EM analysis
and corresponds to the section designated C in Fig. 3. The distribution of synapses is shown in a separate histogram for each dog. Adjacent to each histogram is a photomicrograph, which shows the cytoarchitectonic features of the
cortex from which that distribution was derived. In each histogram, the number
of synapses per 1,000 μ^2 of tissue is presented as a function of cortical depth
(class interval $= 50 \mu$). Table 1 contains the data from which these distributions
were constructed.

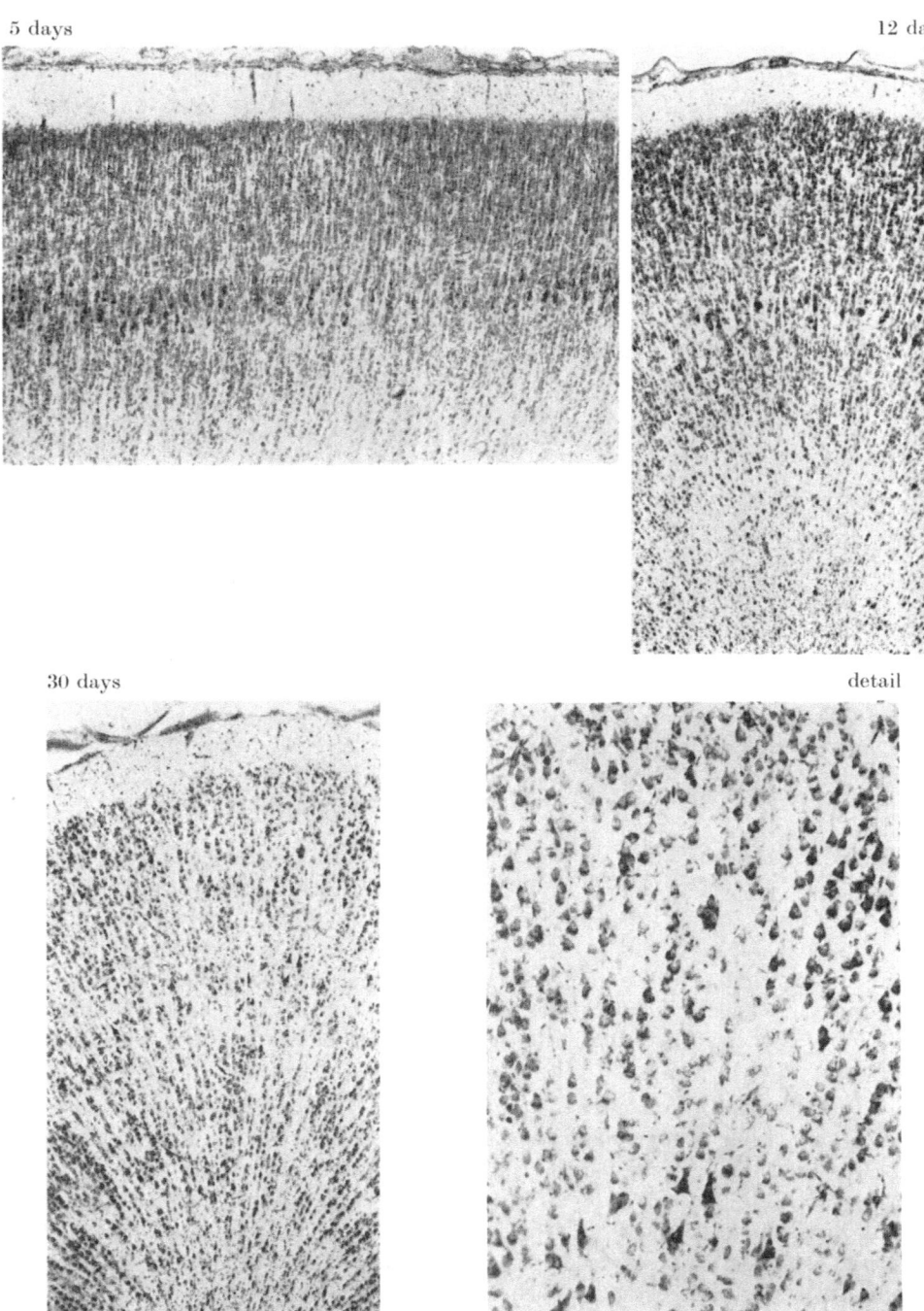

Fig. 16. Somesthetic cortex of dog at selected stages of maturation. The layer of large cells in the young dog can be equated with layer V of the mature dog. Nissl method (Golgi-Cox, destained, methylene blue-Cl). Magn. ×36; detail of 30 day dog at ×100

Table I. Synapses per depth-class — raw data

The table shows the actual number of definite synapses (Grade 1—4) and the number of suspicious appositions (Grade 5—6) in each 50 μ depth-class. For every depth-class, the inspected area of tissue is given. The number of definite synapses in each depth-class is multiplied by the correction factor (1000 ÷ inspected area) to obtain the corrected number of synapses, which is presented in the histograms. (Although some probes were as deep as 1,500 μ, the number of synapses in the deepest depth-classes is not presented because of insufficient data from those depths.)

Depth (μ)	Dog I synapses Grades 1—4	Dog I synapses Grades 5—6	Dog I inspected area (μ²)	Dog I correction factor	Dog II synapses Grades 1—4	Dog II synapses Grades 5—6	Dog II inspected area (μ²)	Dog II correction factor	Dog III synapses Grades 1—4	Dog III synapses Grades 5—6	Dog III inspected area (μ²)	Dog III correction factor
50	30	14	1,026.8	0.97	19	5	1,049	0.95	11	7	455	2.2
100	31	8	1,026.8	0.97	26	3	1,018	0.98	11	2	455	2.2
150	8	7	1,026.8	0.97	12	2	1,018	0.98	2	0	455	2.2
200	5	4	1,026.8	0.97	11	1	953	1.05	2	0	390	2.6
250	7	1	1,026.8	0.97	10	2	1,018	0.98	3	1	455	2.2
300	4	0	1,026.8	0.97	4	3	1,049	0.95	0	1	455	2.2
350	5	2	1,026.8	0.97	3	1	953	1.05	3	2	390	2.6
400	5	1	1,026.8	0.97	5	1	1,018	0.98	3	6	455	2.2
450	12	0	1,026.8	0.97	1	0	1,018	0.98	3	0	455	2.2
500	6	2	615.4	1.62	8	1	1,102	0.91	7	3	390	2.6
550	6	3	656	1.52	9	4	1,488	0.67	6	1	455	2.2
600	13	2	689	1.45	10	6	2,132	0.47	8	3	455	2.2
650	17	1	689	1.45	14	8	2,034	0.49	3	0	390	2.6
700	6	0	656	1.52	12	1	1,093	0.92	13	5	792	1.3
750	16	4	1,050	0.95	15	5	965	1.04	10	4	792	1.3
800	24	6	984	1.02	6	7	965	1.04	9	4	697	1.4
850	17	4	689	1.45	11	10	965	1.04	9	3	337	3.0
900	12	5	689	1.45	27	4	965	1.04	4	1	337	3.0
950	7	4	656	1.52	6	2	965	1.04	3	1	337	3.0
1,000	8	2	689	1.45	16	8	965	1.04	5	0	337	3.0
1,050	10	1	656	1.52	9	3	965	1.04	6	1	307	3.3
1,100	2	4	689	1.45	8	4	997	1.00	3	4	337	3.0
1,150	4	2	689	1.45	17	2	965	1.04	3	1	337	3.0
1,200	2	2	656	1.52	6	5	965	1.04	4	1	337	3.0
1,250	2	0	328	3.05	10	5	965	1.04	0	0	337	3.0
1,300					7	2	965	1.04	4	0	337	3.0
1,350					11	5	965	1.04	2	0	337	3.0
1,400					6	5	965	1.04				

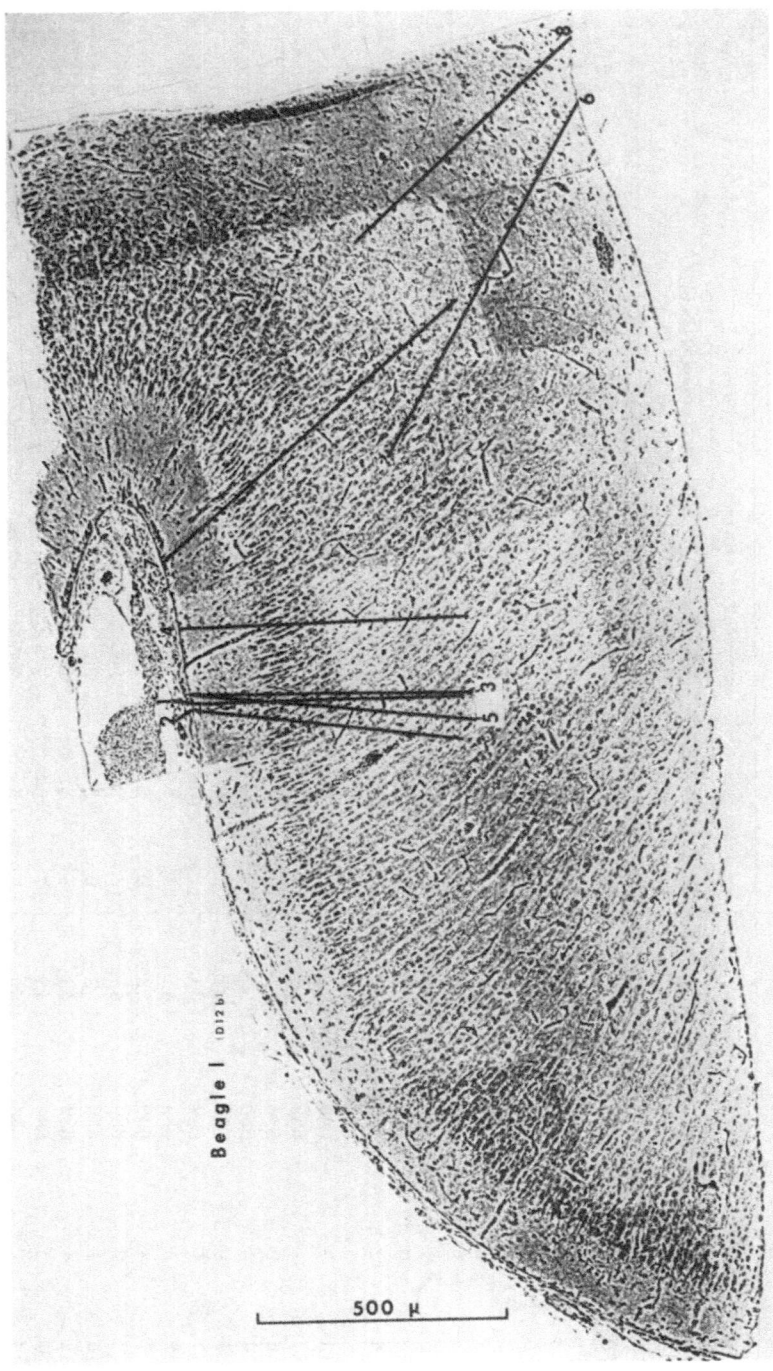

Fig. 17

Beagle II (B 3 b)   Beagle III (B 10 a)

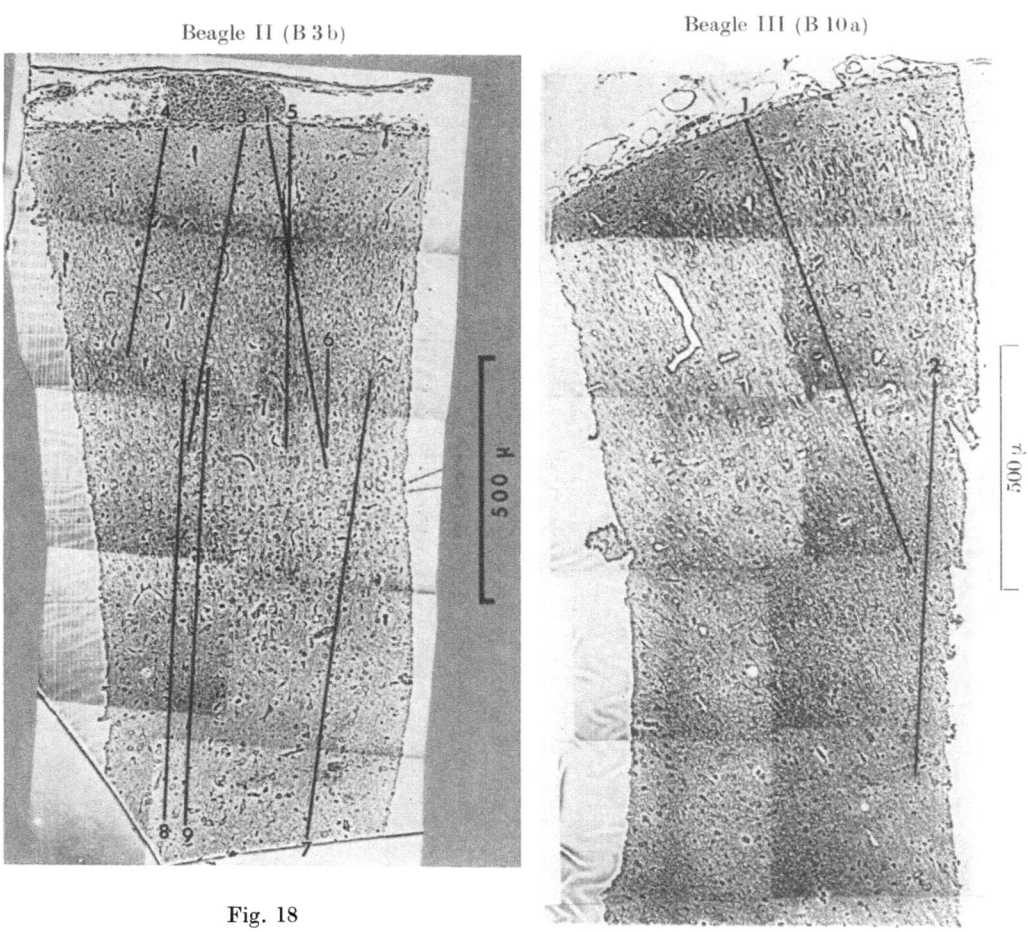

Fig. 18

Fig. 19

Figs. 17—19. Probe locations in cortex from Dogs I, II and III. Shown are phase contrast micrographs of thick sections (equivalent to Fig. 3, C) which are adjacent to the thin sections used for electron microscopic analysis. Each numbered line represents the location of a probe. (Note overlap of superficial and deep probes; this overlap results in a large inspected area. See Table I for correction factors.) Collages; magn. ×70

The synaptic distribution derived from Dog I (Fig. 20) is based on the study of 259 definite synapses (grades 1 to 4) taken from a total inspected area of 20,617 μ^2. Examination of this distribution reveals that certain cortical depths are characterized by high synaptic density, others by low synaptic density. In Dog I there is a very high synaptic density in cortical layer I. There is also a peak of synaptic density at the depth of the large cell layer (600 μ) and another peak lying at a depth of 800 μ. Cortical loci in which synapses are rare lie just below layer I and at the lower border of the large cell layer.

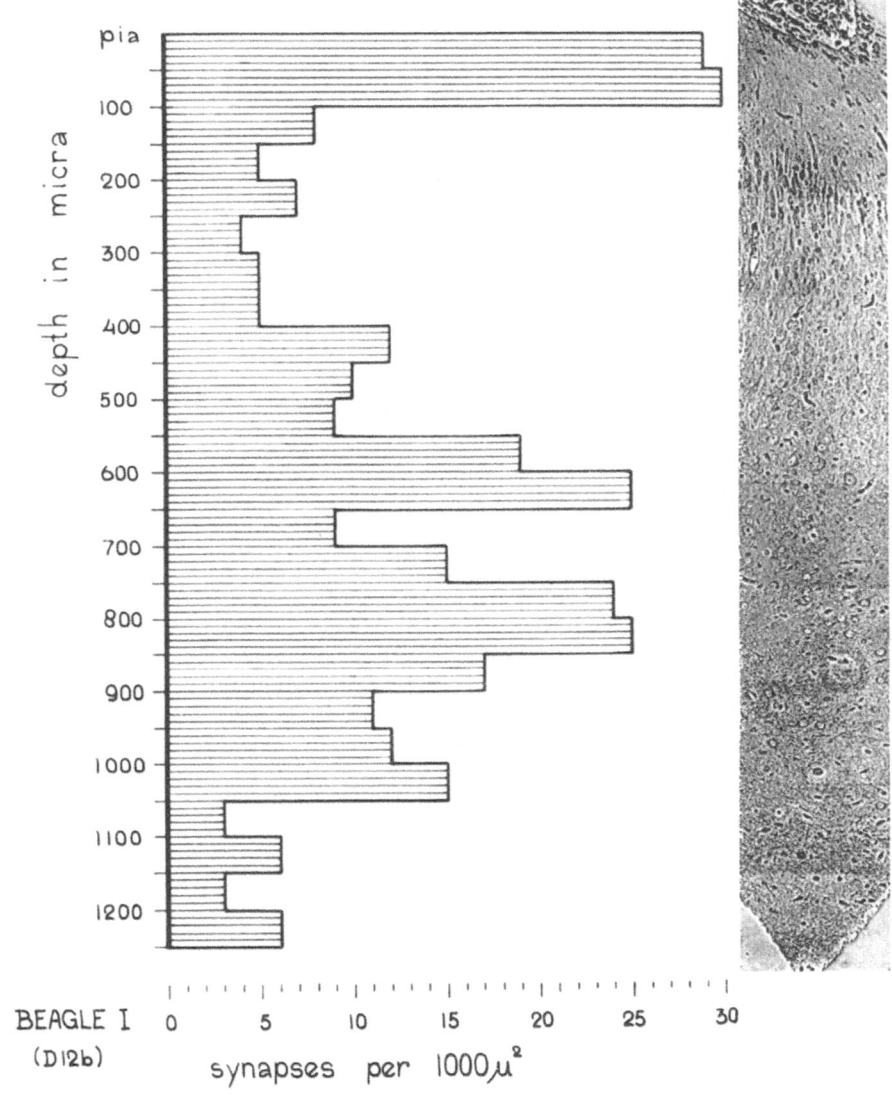

Fig. 20. Distribution of synaptic contacts as a function of cortical depth—Dog I. Class interval = 50 μ. For each depth-class, the number of synapses is expressed per 1,000 μ² of tissue area. Shown on the right is a strip of cortex selected from a thick section in the series used for analysis. The magnification of the micrograph (×100) conforms to the depth scale of the histogram

The distribution of synapses from Dog II is based upon 301 definite synapses and derived from the inspection of 30,835 μ². The histogram (Fig. 21) reveals bands of high and low synaptic density that bear the same relationship to cortical cytoarchitectonics as that seen in Dog I. High magnification views of layer I and of the large cell layer more clearly demonstrate the spatial relationships between the peaks of synaptic density and the cytoarchitectonic pattern of the cortex in Dog II (Fig. 22).

The cortex of a third animal was analyzed to support the preceding results and to determine how closely the above distributions might be approached by using a minimum amount of data. (This question will be of practical significance to us in attempting, with few data, to ascertain what other stages of development may be the most fruitful to study in detail.) The synaptic distribution of Dog III is based upon only one probe through the superficial cortex and one probe through the deep cortex (cf. Fig. 19). In an inspected area of 11,613 μ^2, 137 definite synapses were found. Although based on insufficient data, the histogram of this animal (Fig. 23) reveals synaptic peaks that are remarkably consistent with those of Dogs I and II. This result justifies the use of a single probe to select the optimal specimens for more systematic analysis.

Identification of Postsynaptic Elements. The locations of high synaptic density indicate where in cortex neurons interact. These data do not indicate the identity of the neurons which interact. Distant presynaptic cells may be found by using degeneration methods; nearby (intracortical) presynaptic cells may be identified by use of a rapid Golgi method for axons. The postsynaptic elements (dendrites and perikarya) may be found by a Golgi-Cox analysis of synapse-dense regions. In this part of our study we have attempted to identify only the postsynaptic elements.

In Golgi-Cox impregnated sections of newborn cortex, we have sought cells whose receptive (i.e. dendritic) surfaces lie within a region of high synaptic density. Amongst these cells must be neurons which provide the postsynaptic elements of that region. The cytoarchitectonic relations of Golgi-Cox impregnated cells are determined, in our material, by reference to immediately adjacent sections which are stained by a Nissl method[9].

Several cell types (Fig. 24) have receptive elements which lie in the synapse-dense region of layer I. Most striking of these are the Retzius-Cajal cells, which can be found only up to about 12 days of age (in dog). We have observed that Retzius-Cajal cells may be located anywhere within layer I of newborn cortex and are especially prevalent at the site of developing sulci. There also is a prominent group of small, immature pyramidal cells, the somata of which lie in layer II, about 200 to 300 μ beneath the pia. The apical dendrites of these pyramids penetrate into layer I and terminate within the region of high synaptic density in a small bouquet often possessing a few gemmules. The basal dendrites of most of these pyramids have not yet appeared. Other small neurons lie entirely within layer I, but these are not common.

In the synapse-dense region associated with the layer of large cells, there are pyramids of all sizes plus cells which may be young stellate cells or stellate pyramids. Many cells whose perikarya lie just above the layer of large cells are characterized by basal dendrite systems that are extensively branched and possess gemmules (Fig. 25); the apical dendrites of these cells rarely have a

---

9 The depths shown in Figs. 24 and 25 are measured directly on the sections from which the cells were taken. These measured depths may not be precisely juxtaposed with the depths derived from the plastic-embedded material due to (slight) differential shrinkage.

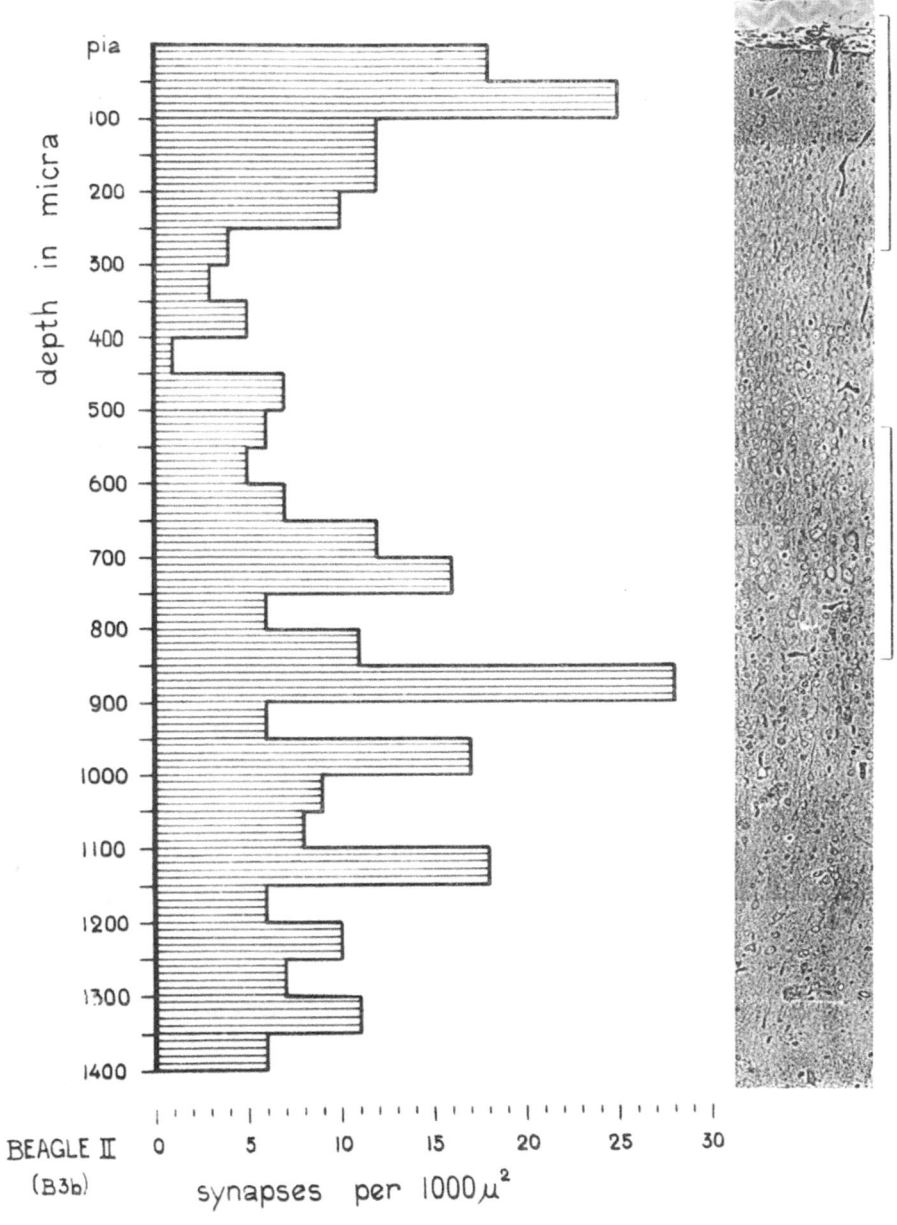

Fig. 21. Distribution of synaptic contacts as a function of cortical depth--Dog II. For details see legend of Fig. 20. Brackets indicate location of high magnification views shown in Fig. 22

bouquet or spines, but terminate bluntly, often beneath layer I. The elaborate basal dendrites of these cells lie in the synapse-dense region associated with the layer of large cells.

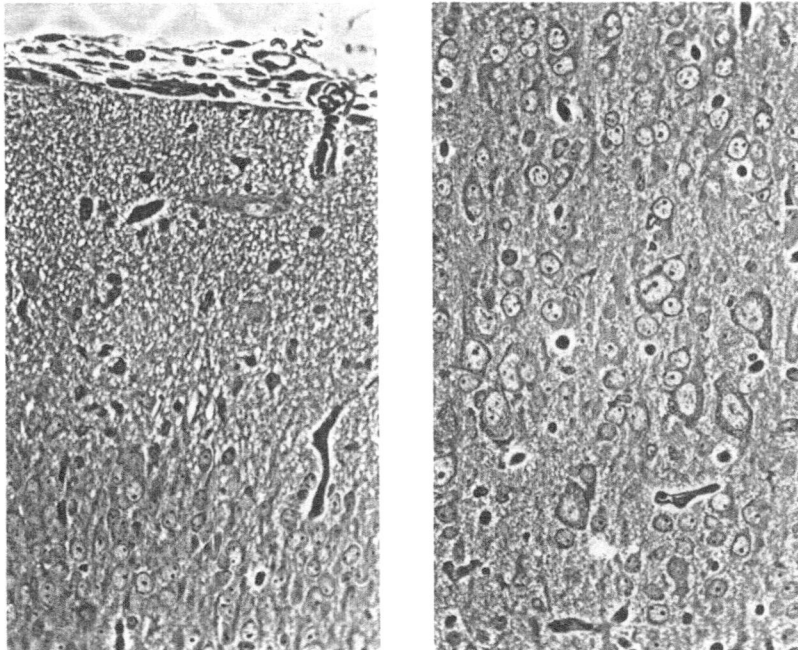

Fig. 22. Details from micrograph in Fig. 21, cortex of Dog II. These phase contrast photo-micrographs show layer I (on left) and large cell layer (on right). Magn. ×280

We have judged the maturity of a neuron on the basis of its dendrite morpho-logy. Our criteria for estimating the maturity of a dendrite are the number and extent of its branches and the density of its spines. Our observations in newborn dog confirm that, with respect to basal dendrites, the deeper cortical neurons (e.g., somata at 600 μ) are more mature than superficially located neurons. Furthermore, the superficial pyramidal cells have apical dendrites that are more mature than their basal dendrites; the deeper neurons are character-ized by greater maturity of their basal dendrites as compared with their apical dendrites. Thus, Cajal's principle that apical dendrites mature earlier than basal dendrites is not of general validity (cf. Fig. 25).

The results of our Golgi-analysis lead to the generalization that dendrites which lie in synapse-dense regions are more mature than dendrites in synapse-poor regions. However, our data are derived from only a qualitative study of Golgi-Cox material. They are presented as a sample of our initial steps in attempting to define the elements which interact in a synapse-dense region of immature cortex.

Discussion

Our specific aim in this initial study was to find the locations of synapses in immature cortex. The distribution of synapses was analyzed as a function of cortical depth. Since the early growth of dendrites first occurs at preferential

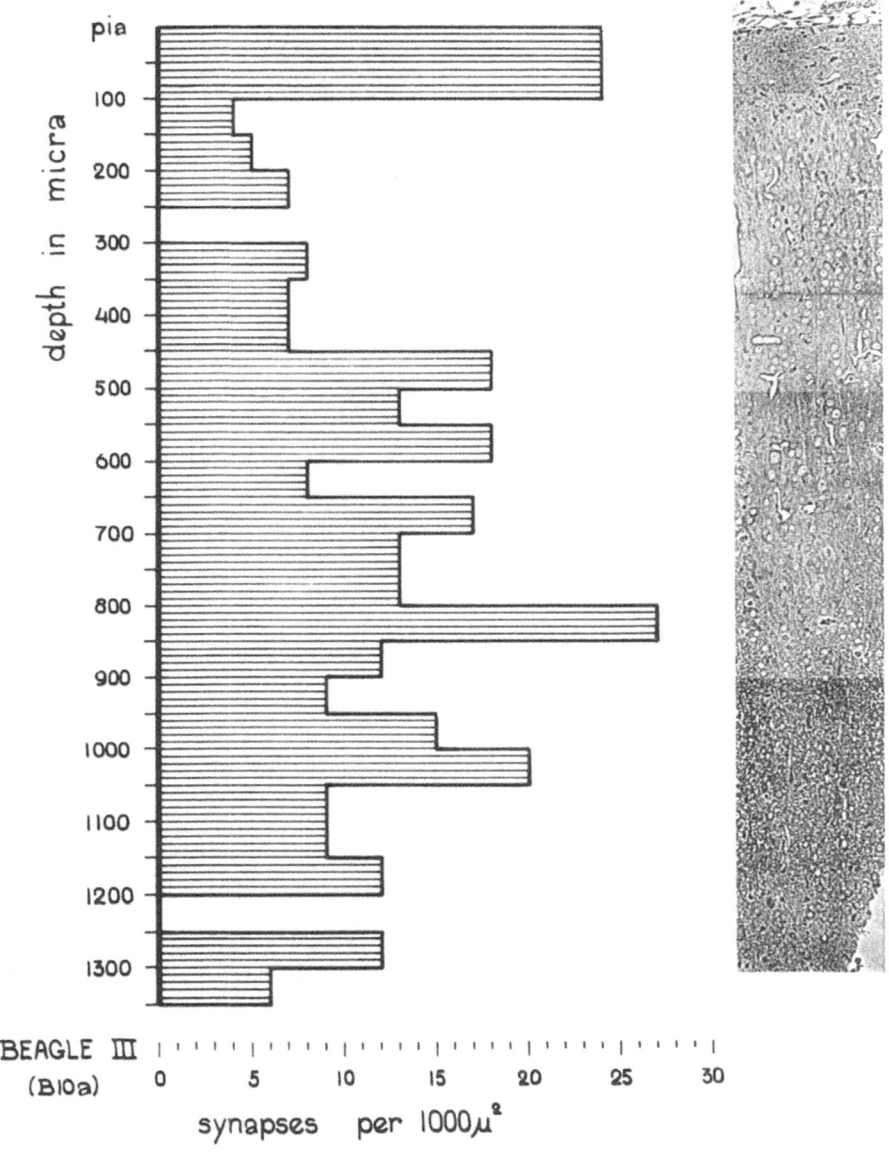

Fig. 23. Distribution of synaptic contacts as a function of cortical depth—Dog III. Data are derived from only one deep and one superficial probe. For details see legend of Fig. 20

depths within the cortex, it seemed not unreasonable to expect that synaptic formation might also occur at preferential depths.

In order to find the distribution of synapses, a method was adopted for making radial probes through the cortex, using the electron microscope. It is necessary to use the higher resolution of electron optics in order to demonstrate, with cer-

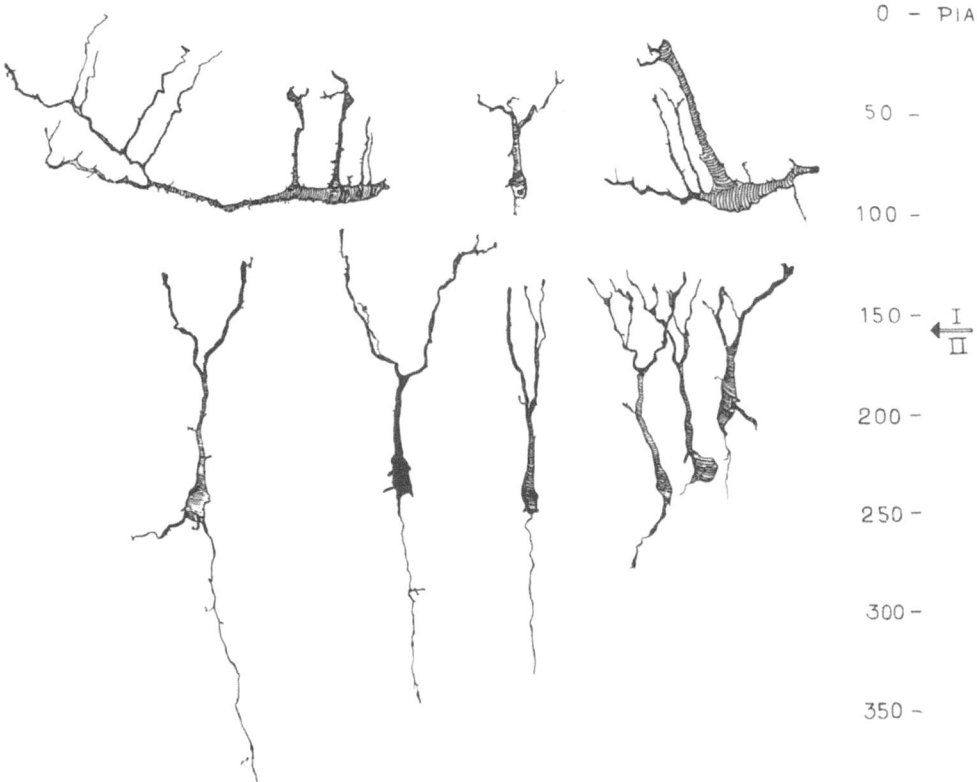

Fig. 24. The most probable postsynaptic elements of layer I (newborn dog, somesthetic cortex). Camera lucida drawings of Golgi-Cox impregnated neurons. Apical dendrites of many superficial pyramids (not shown) terminate within 50 μ of the pial surface. Numbers denote depth (in micra) beneath pia. Arrow indicates interface between layers I and II. Magn. ×270

tainty, the presence of synaptic contacts. The locations of cortical synapses may be inferred but not demonstrated by light microscopic methods. For example, the light microscopic demonstration of the presence of postsynaptic elements suggests but does not demonstrate the existence of synaptic contacts (Van der Loos, 1968).

The distributions of synaptic contacts in Dogs I and II may be juxtaposed for direct comparison (Fig. 26, see legend). The histograms demonstrate that synaptic contacts are neither evenly nor randomly distributed through cortical depth. The synapses are grouped in definite strata which are consistently related to cytoarchitectonic layers. The bands of high synaptic density, designated A, B, and C in Fig. 26, we call "synaptic strata". We refer to the synaptic organization of the cortex as "synaptoarchitectonics".

The functional significance of a synaptic stratum is determined by its role in cortical circuitry. This role cannot be known until the pre- and postsynaptic elements are identified. Knowing the location of a synaptic stratum permits us to go directly to the other elements of circuitry, i. e., the two elements which meet

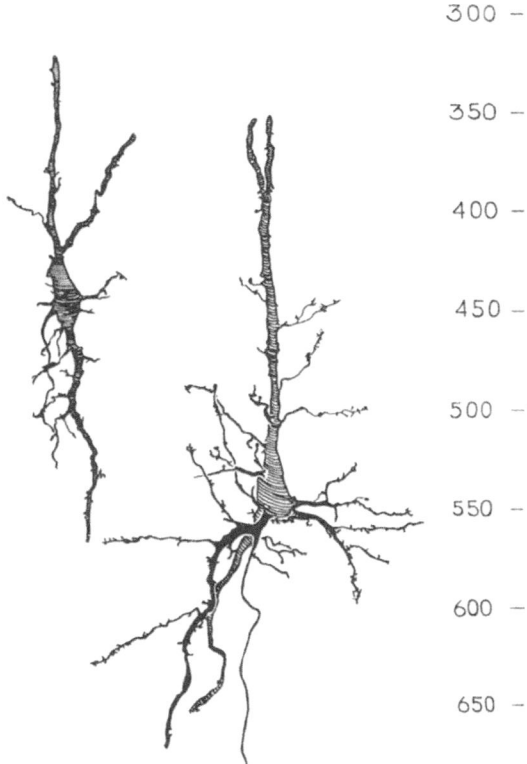

Fig. 25. Neurons which lie just above the layer of large cells (newborn dog, somesthetic cortex). Camera lucida drawing of two representative neurons impregnated by a Golgi-Cox method. Basal dendrites of pyramidal cell (at right) are at a depth of high synaptic density; gemmules are numerous. Apical dendrite is short and relatively unbranched. Compare apical and basal dendrite maturity with that of more superficial pyramids (Fig. 24). Numbers denote depth (in micra) beneath pia. Magn. ×270

and interact at each synaptic junction. We have used Golgi material from neonatal cortex to identify those neurons whose receptive surfaces lie within each synaptic stratum. It was found that the most likely postsynaptic elements of synaptic stratum A (in layer I) are the Retzius-Cajal cells and the apical dendrites of small pyramids which have their perikarya in layer II. The deeper synapses, which make up synaptic strata B and C, lie in close relation to the layer of large cells (layer V). Amongst the most likely postsynaptic elements of synaptic stratum B are the abundant and relatively mature basal dendrites of pyramidal neurons which lie immediately superficial to the large cell layer (Fig. 25); the basal dendrites of these pyramids lie in the region which later becomes layer IV. The postsynaptic elements of synaptic stratum C may include the basal dendrites of the large cells of layer V.

It should be emphasized that the morphology of Golgi impregnated immature neurons does not necessarily lead to the proper adult classification of these cells;

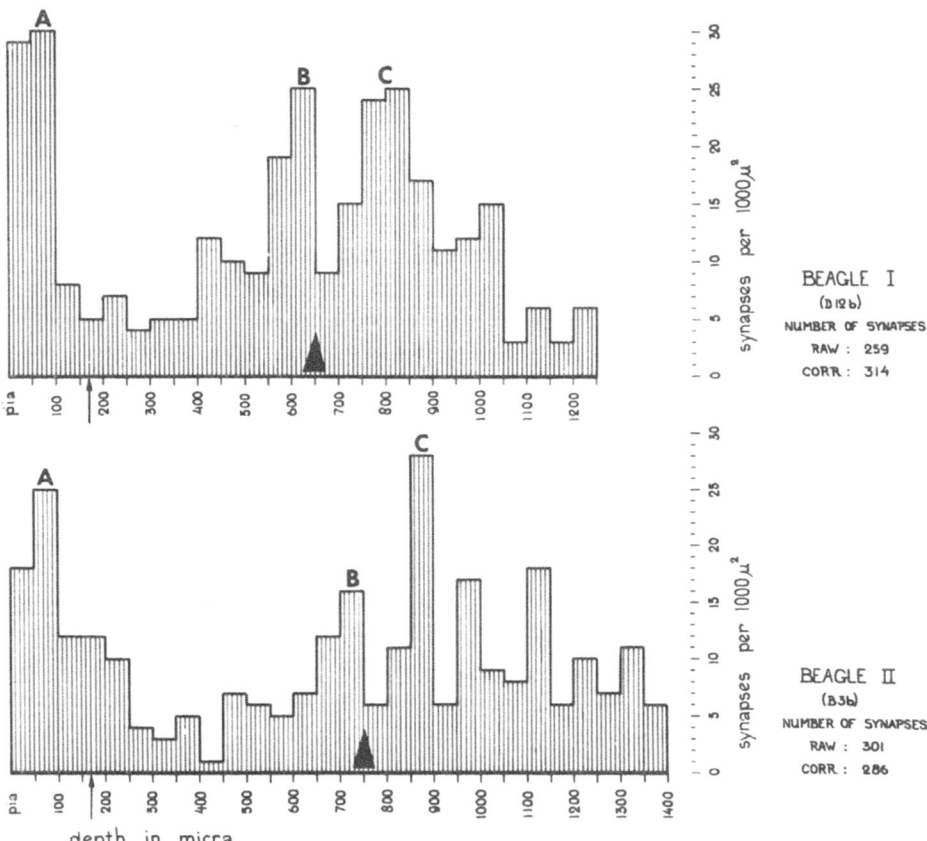

Fig. 26. Synapse distributions in somesthetic cortex from Dogs I and II. Histograms from Figs. 20 and 21 are juxtaposed for direct comparison. Arrow points to interface between layers I and II. △ indicates location of layer of large cells. Peaks of highest synaptic density— synaptic strata — are designated by letters A, B and C

for example, young pyramids may become stellate pyramids, and the fate of Retzius-Cajal cells is unknown. Quantitative Golgi studies are necessary to identify more comprehensively the postsynaptic elements in each synaptic stratum. The identification of postsynaptic neurons is complicated by the fact that dendrites within one synaptic stratum may stem from perikarya which lie in other layers. Furthermore, a neuron which extends its dendrites over many layers may receive input from multiple synaptic strata. The definitive identification of postsynaptic neurons would be simplified if we knew where, on the young neuron, synapses are found; we plan to obtain these data from a separate electron microscopic study of Golgi-impregnated neurons.

We do not have morphologic evidence, in the newborn, that permits us to identify the cell bodies of origin of the presynaptic elements. In a subsequent section, we shall speculate about the source of input to the synaptic strata on the basis of physiologic information.

In each of the neonatal dogs studied, two well-delineated strata of low synaptic density have been found (Fig. 26). One is a broad band that is consistently associated with the region of high cell density just beneath layer I. This cell layer of the cortex appears to be the primordium of layer II and, perhaps, of part of layer III. The other synapse-poor region is a narrow band located at the lower border of the large cell layer (i. e. layer V), and it separates synaptic strata B and C.

What factors are responsible for synapse-poor strata in young cortices? Potential pre- and postsynaptic elements may be present in these strata but may not have yet made contact. Alternatively, axons destined to form the presynaptic elements may not have yet grown into the strata under consideration. Also, a layer of cortex may be densely packed with somata which possess rudimentary dendritic systems; virtually no dendrites would be available as postsynaptic elements in such a layer (axo-somatic synapses are extremely rare).

We cannot yet determine which factors may be responsible for the two synapse-poor bands described above. The more superficial synapse-poor band lies in a locus characterized by dense packing of cells with minimal development of basal dendrites (Figs. 22 and 24). In contrast, the deeper synapse-poor band, at the lower border of layer V, is a region of low perikaryon density which is traversed by a moderate number of neuronal processes. The different composition of these two strata indicates that low synaptic density is not merely a consequence of high perikaryal density associated with unavailability of neuropil. Moreover, inspection of the overall relationship between synapse distribution and cytoarchitectonics (Figs. 20, 21, 23) reveals that the relationship between synaptic density and perikaryal density is a poorly fitting one.

The association of synaptic strata with bands of mature dendrites is important in considering mechanisms of neuronal growth. The strata of greatest synaptic density, designated A, B and C, correspond in location to pale bands which are seen in Nissl-stained sections of immature cortex[10]. As noted in the Introduction, Lorente de Nó (1933) recognized that the pale bands represent strata of early maturing dendrites. In the present study we have demonstrated that indeed strata of high synaptic density coincide with strata containing numerous mature dendrites. This spatial relationship suggests that dendrite maturation may be causally related to synapse formation. For example, functioning synapses may exert a trophic influence on dendrite growth. Conversely, dendrite maturity may be a prerequisite for synapse formation.

It will be of particular interest, in future studies, to follow strata of high synaptic density back into prenatal life and to follow strata of low synaptic density forward into maturity. In this way, we may determine the temporal and spatial patterns of synapse formation and the concurrent patterns of dendrite growth. Thus, the synaptic strata are static morphologic phenomena that will be useful in studying the formation of neuronal circuits. In immature cortex a synaptic stratum may represent a specific functional system with a single type of input, as yet "uncontaminated" by other inputs. Hence, in young cortex, it may be feasible to isolate functionally pure interneuronal circuits by both morphologic and physio-

---

10 Plastic sections of 1 μ thickness are too thin to reveal the pale (perikaryon-poor) bands, which are best seen in Nissl-stained sections of 20—30 μ thickness (cf. Fig. 16 — 5 days).

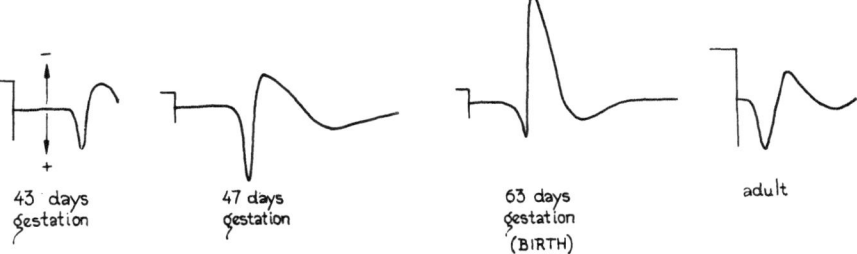

43 days
gestation

47 days
gestation

63 days
gestation
(BIRTH)

adult

Fig. 27. Surface potentials recorded from primary somesthetic cortex, evoked by tactile stimulation. Data are shown from four ages. Polarity: positive down. Calibration bars: vertical, 100 μV; horizontal, 25 msec. (Taken from paper in preparation)

logic methods. Caution should be exercised in making conclusions about adult circuitry from neonatal data. Patterns of interneuronal organization may be different in young and in adult cortices since neurons may move to other locations, and synapses which are present at birth may not be permanent.

A fundamental question remains: is the existence of synaptic strata a general phenomenon of cortical organization? We do not yet know if synaptic strata exist anywhere in mature neocortex or in regions of neonatal cortex other than the primary somesthetic area.

Another problem of interpretation of the data remains unresolved. In the newborn, the border between cortex and "white" matter can be delineated by light microscopic examination and lies at a depth of approximately 1,000 μ (cf. Fig. 14). Inspection at high magnification reveals neurons scattered through the intermediate zone from ependyma to cortex. Our deepest electron microscopic probes reveal synapses down to 1,500 μ beneath the pia, which is as deep as we have inspected. These "subcortical" synapses may be in regions destined to become cortex, or they may be on neurons which are migrating through the "white" matter. In the latter case, the following question arises: where do migrating neurons first acquire synapses? Further studies are indicated to analyze the synaptic distribution from cortex to ependyma.

An analysis of the relationship between electrical phenomena of the cortex and the structures which generate those phenomena is of value for the understanding of functional organization of cortical circuitry. The synaptic strata introduced in this paper can be meaningfully related to certain electrophysiologic properties of neonatal cortex.

Stimulation of cutaneous sensory receptors produces a (slow) electrical response which can be recorded from the cortical surface. The wave-form of the response undergoes a series of characteristic changes during ontogenesis (Fig. 27). In mid-fetal life, this response is characterized by a very long latency and is predominantly surface-positive (dog: Molliver, in prep.; sheep: Molliver, 1967). In later fetal stages, the positive wave remains and is followed by a negative wave which gradually increases in amplitude as the fetus matures. At the time of birth (dog: Molliver, in prep.; cat: Oeconomos and Scherrer, 1953) the negative wave has become very large in amplitude, and it dominates the evoked response (Fig. 27). This predominant negativity of the evoked response during an intermediate period of maturation is a well established characteristic of primary sensory cortices in many species (dog: Molliver, in prep.; cat: Ellingson and Wilcott, 1960; Marty, 1962; Oeconomos and Scherrer, 1953; Purpura, 1961a; rabbit: Hunt and Goldring, 1951; Marty, 1962; sheep: Meyerson and Persson, 1969; Molliver, 1967; human: Ellingson, 1960). During subsequent postnatal development, the amplitude of the surface-negative wave gradually diminishes until the evoked response reaches its mature configuration (by 21 days of age in dog): an initially and predominantly positive wave (Fig. 27).

In mature animals, the electrical potentials recorded from the surface of the cortex could arise from multiple patterns of neuronal activity. Simultaneous recording of cortical surface potentials and of the activity of single neurons has been used by several investigators to analyze the correlation between these events. Evidence has emerged (Amassian, Waller and Macy, 1964; Calvet, Calvet and Scherrer, 1964; Creutzfeldt, Watanabe and Lux, 1966; Mountcastle, Davies and Berman, 1957; Purpura, 1959) in support of the view that evoked surface potentials are usually the sign of current flow associated with postsynaptic potentials in neurons which are arranged in an orderly (laminar) pattern (Mountcastle and Poggio, 1968). A strong, temporal relationship has been found between the initial, positive phase of the adult evoked potential and the excitatory postsynaptic potentials (EPSP's) of neurons lying deep in the cortex (e. g., Amassian, Waller and Macy, 1964; Calvet, Calvet and Scherrer, 1964; Mountcastle, Davies and Berman, 1957). Yet, because of the complexity of synaptic organization in adult cortex, the definitive relationship between surface potentials and synaptic events remains obscure.

In immature cortex, the problem of relating synaptic activity to surface potentials is simplified by the relative paucity of synapses and by their stratiform arrangement. Thus, in a young animal, a large cortical surface potential may be generated by semi-synchronous activity of the postsynaptic elements within a single synaptic stratum. We propose that the predominantly negative evoked cortical response of the newborn dog (Fig. 27) is produced by EPSP's in synaptic stratum A, which lies in layer I. The most likely postsynaptic elements in layer I of neonatal cortex have been described above (cf. Fig. 24), i. e., apical dendrites of pyramidal cells with somata in layers II—III, and the Retzius-Cajal cells. The pyramidal cells referred to have apical dendrite bouquets which lie in synaptic stratum A and which possess some gemmules; the perikarya of these cells lie in a region of low synaptic density (200—300 μ beneath the pia) and their basal dendrites are rudimentary. Thus, synapses upon these cells must be largely restricted to the terminal segment of the apical dendrites. Excitatory synapses of synaptic stratum A would produce membrane depolarization in the apical dendrites of these neurons. Depolarization restricted to the ad-pial portion of such a cell would establish an electrical dipole, with the soma region positive and the apical dendrite negative. An array of such dipoles, with their positive poles oriented toward the ventricle and their negative poles oriented toward the pia, would present a large negative charge to an electrode placed on the pial surface. Many of these apical dendrites terminate within 50 μ of the pia.

The Retzius-Cajal cells, which lie in layer I, may also be postsynaptic elements of synaptic stratum A. Synapses upon these cells have not yet been demonstrated definitively. Depolarizing postsynaptic potentials in these large cells would present a negative charge to a relatively small electrode placed on the pial surface just above the site of depolarization. These unique neurons have numerous vertical dendrite branches that ascend and terminate in small expansions under the pia (Figs. 2 and 24). These vertical branches, or the extracellular fluid around them, may possibly provide low impedance paths from a depolarized region of the cell directly to the pia and thus enhance the surface-negative potential. The Retzius-Cajal cells are numerous in the cortex only during the time that the surface-negative potential is prominent.

Inhibitory postsynaptic potentials (IPSP's) must also be considered as possible contributors to evoked surface responses. IPSP's generated deep in the cortex could enhance the surface negativity, but we deem it unlikely that such IPSP's contribute substantially to the prominent surface-negative response of the newborn.

As noted above, we do not have morphologic data that permit us to locate the perikarya of origin of the presynaptic elements of cortical synapses. However, the available physiologic evidence permits us to make some (tentative) hypotheses about the nature of synaptic input to the immature cortex. The observation that, in somesthetic cortex of newborn dog, slow surface potentials are evoked by stimulation of cutaneous receptors indicates that there is a functioning somesthetic pathway from the periphery to the cortex. The prominent negativity of the evoked response indicates that depolarization of neuronal elements close to the pial surface is produced as a result of synaptic impingement of the afferent pathway (directly or through other cortical neurons). That this afferent pathway is part of the specific afferent system (versus generalized) is supported by the following evidence. The evoked surface-negative response of the newborn dog is localized to a small area of primary somesthetic cortex (Molliver, in prep.). There is a reproducible topologic relationship between the cortical location of the negative evoked response and the location of the peripheral area stimulated. During the course of development, there is a gradual and continuous transition from the negative evoked response of the newborn to the primary evoked response of the adult. In newborn cat (Purpura, 1961a) and rabbit (Farber, 1968) the characteristic surface-negative response is evoked in primary sensory cortex by electrical stimulation of *specific* thalamic relay nuclei. On the basis of the foregoing arguments, we propose that synaptic stratum A, in the newborn, contains axon terminals of neurons which are part of the specific somesthetic pathway.

It is likely that the synapses of layer IV in the newborn (synaptic stratum B) represent terminals of the specific thalamocortical axons, as is generally believed to be true in adult primary projection cortices (Cajal, 1900; Hubel and Wiesel, 1969; Lorente de Nó, 1938; Nauta, 1954; Poljak, 1927). We as yet have but little evidence to support that hypothesis in the neonatal period. In the newborn dog and cat, single neurons in both deep and superficial cortical regions are driven by cutaneous stimulation (Molliver, in prep.). Similar findings were reported in sheep at an equivalent developmental stage (Meyerson and Persson, 1969). Thus, somesthetic input must impinge, directly or indirectly, on deep as well as on superficial neurons.

Postsynaptic potentials in deep neurons do not necessarily have a predominant influence on the wave-form of potentials recorded from the cortical surface of the newborn[11]. These deeper lying synapses are over ten times the distance from the recording electrode as are the active elements of layer I. (If the cortical impedance were uniform throughout, the effect of a charge upon a distant electrode would be inversely proportional to the distance of that charge from the electrode.)

The proposed relationship between the surface-negative potentials of immature cortex and postsynaptic potentials in layer I is in accord with earlier proposals (Bernhard, Kolmodin and Meyerson, 1967; Marty, 1962; Molliver, 1967; Purpura, 1961 a; Verley, 1965). However, those earlier hypotheses, based primarily on physiologic observations, were tenuous in that they were based upon insufficient morphologic evidence[12]. Our demonstration of a stratum of high synaptic density in layer I and, beneath it, a broad band of very low synaptic density makes the proposed relationship highly probable. The evidence presented here provides a morphologic basis for the existence of neuronal circuits which can generate a surface negativity. The same evidence makes it highly improbable that postsynaptic potentials in layers II or III could produce the large surface-negative response of the newborn dog.

The surface-negative response of the neonate represents but a single stage in the development of the evoked cortical response.

Our morphologic studies have been restricted to the newborn period, and we do not have evidence that permits a meaningful analysis of the structural basis for the evoked cortical response in older animals[13]. The existence of a different response characteristic (surface positivity) early in fetal life, suggests that in that period a different (and relatively simple) pattern of synapse distribution may exist. Therefore, it would be relevant to analyze the synaptoarchitectonic pattern of the fetal dog at 40 to 45 days of gestation. As a guide to our future studies of prenatal cortex we have formulated a working hypothesis which relates the

---

11 EPSP's generated deep in the cortex may be used to explain two minor features of the neonatal evoked response. (1) The evoked surface-negative response is always preceded by a small, positive wave (Molliver, 1967). (2) The application of GABA to the cortical surface (presumedly blocking EPSP's in superficial dendrites) is followed by disappearance of the surface-negative response, and the subsequent appearance of an evoked surface-positive response (Purpura, 1961 b). The frequent spontaneous appearance of surface-positive waves in the EEG of newborn rabbit (Garma, 1966) may also be related to deep EPSP's.

12 The relationship between the surface-negative evoked response of neonatal cortex and activity in "superficial axodendritic pathways" proposed by Purpura (1961 a) (p. 618, 651) and by Purpura, Shofer, Housepian and Noback (1964, p. 200) was based largely upon morphologic data from both a Golgi analysis (Noback and Purpura, 1961) and an electron microscopic study (Voeller, Pappas and Purpura, 1963) of immature feline neocortex. Synapses were demonstrated on large apical dendrite trunks (Voeller, Pappas and Purpura, 1963) *beneath* layer I (see Introduction), but no synapses were demonstrated on the apical dendrite bouquets within layer I. This distribution of synapses over the neuronal surface cannot be used to explain the relationship proposed by Purpura, because EPSP's in apical dendrite *trunks* of superficial pyramids would produce either no net surface potential or a positive-negative sequence. The generation of the prominent surface-negative wave would require EPSP's in the apical dendrite bouquets in layer I.

13 Fox (1968), in a study of immature dogs, has attempted to correlate morphologic phenomena of cortical maturation with both the development of evoked potentials and the development of social behavior. Data taken from these operationally different realms were juxtaposed, and the mechanisms by which the phenomena may be related to one another were not postulated.

evoked potentials characteristic of prenatal life to synaptic strata which may be present at the same time.

It was shown above that, in the newborn, neurons with perikarya at an approximate depth of 600 μ beneath the pia have well developed basal dendrites which lie within synaptic stratum B. These basal dendrites, which possess many gemmules, appear significantly more mature than the postsynaptic elements (apical dendrite bouquets) of layer I (cf. Figs. 24 and 25). It is thus probable that the deep basal dendrites engage in synaptic contacts earlier than the apical dendrites of layer I. We propose that synaptic stratum B was formed earlier in ontogenesis than synaptic stratum A.

In the newborn, the deep neurons with relatively mature basal dendrites in synaptic stratum B have immature apical dendrites which lie in a band of low synaptic density (Fig. 25).

Hence, synapses on these neurons must be largely restricted to the basal dendrites—in the newborn and certainly in the fetus. Therefore, we predict that in fetal cortex at about 45 days of gestation the only synapses present are on basal dendrites of relatively deep neurons. This proposal that the earliest synapses are formed deep in the cortex is consistent with the principle of Vignal that neuronal maturation, judged by basal dendrite development, begins deep in the cortex[14].

Thus, excitatory synaptic input to the cortex of a fetal dog (about 45 days gestation) may produce depolarization of only the basal dendrites of deep pyramids. Basal dendrite depolarization in one of these neurons would produce an asymmetrical charge distribution, i. e., a dipole, with the basal dendrites electro-negative and the apical dendrite positive. A layer of such polarized cells, oriented with their positive poles toward the pia, would present a positive charge to a surface electrode. According to this hypothetical mechanism, the evoked surface-positive response of fetal dogs is produced by EPSP's deep in the cortex.

In fetal sheep (Molliver, 1967) the earliest somesthetic evoked response is also a surface-positive wave. It was postulated that this positive wave is the sign of excitatory postsynaptic potentials deep in the cortex. An alternative explanation was proposed by Bernhard, Kolmodin and Meyerson (1967): a positive wave at the cortical surface "signals depolarization of the afferent presynaptic terminals" which do not yet engage in functioning synaptic contacts. This latter hypothesis is in agreement with the theory (Bishop and Clare, 1953; Eccles, 1951; Landau and Clare, 1956; Marshall, Talbot and Ades, 1943; Perl and Whitlock, 1955) that a highly synchronous volley of impulses in numerous thalamocortical axons (produced by electrical stimulation of the thalamus) may result in a brief surface-positive potential. However, when natural cutaneous stimulation is applied, no component of afferent fiber activity can be demonstrated in the evoked cortical surface potential (Amassian, Waller and Macy, 1964; Eccles, 1951; Marshall,

---

14 The early development of dendrites and synapses deep in the cortex appears to be consistent with the phenomenon that the deepest cortical layers contain the earliest formed— and therefore the oldest—neurons (Angevine and Sidman, 1961). However, there is no direct evidence that the neurons which are the first to form are the first to mature. Moreover, the early formation of apical dendrites of superficial neurons appears to be in conflict with a strict relationship between the age of the individual nerve cell and its maturation.

Talbot and Ades, 1943; Perl and Whitlock, 1955). Furthermore, the extremely long duration (dog: 40 msec, sheep: 80 msec) of the fetal surface positive response —evoked by tactile stimulation of a small cutaneous point—could only with difficulty be attributed to impulse conduction in a small number of presynaptic corticopetal afferents.

In a recent important study of fetal sheep, Meyerson and Persson (1969) have attempted to relate the activity of single neurons to the cortical surface response evoked by tactile stimulation. At the developmental stage in which the surface response was positive, evoked unit activity could be recorded only from subcortical locations (at 64 days gestation). They concluded that the (fetal) surface-positive wave resulted from subcortical unit activity in afferent nerve fibers, and that synapses had not yet been established between afferent fibers and cortical neurons.

Our interpretation of their data leads us to a quite different conclusion, for the following reasons. First, it is extraordinarily difficult to record from single neurons in the cortex of small fetuses: the skull and cortex are physically unstable; neurons are small, densely packed, and extremely fragile; and impulses are infrequent. Therefore, in fetal cortex, the failure to record impulses from single neurons does not constitute evidence that cortical neurons are not synaptically driven. Moreover, it is possible that functioning synapses may produce postsynaptic potentials in neurons that can not yet generate impulses. Secondly, the subcortical impulses, recorded by those investigators, do not necessarily arise from afferent fibers, but may, in fact, represent postsynaptic impulse generation in neurons which are migrating toward the cortex. We have observed both neurons and synapses in the subcortical zone of neonatal dog (cf. above).

We conclude that the evidence presented by Meyerson and Persson does not conflict with our hypothesis that the prenatal surface-positive response arises from EPSP's deep in the cortex. In fact, our hypothesis is supported by their observation (at 70 days gestation) that neuronal impulses first appear in the deepest layers of the cortex, when the evoked response is still predominantly surface-positive and the ensuing negative phase is relatively small. We have no experimental basis for rejecting what we deem less likely alternatives, namely that the surface-positive response may be produced either by depolarization of presynaptic afferent fibers or by hyperpolarizing PSP's in layer I. Due to the difficulties in recording from single neurons in fetal cortex, this physiologic problem must be approached by means of a more sensitive, morphologic technique. Hence, we plan to conduct a synaptoarchitectonic analysis of fetal cortex at the age at which the surface-positive response is dominant. If a single stratum of synapses is found, we would conclude that postsynaptic activity in that stratum may produce the surface-positive response. If no synapses are found, then the surface response must be attributed to activity of afferent fibers.

The evoked potentials of immature cortex are not only of value in formulating the functional significance of synaptic strata; they also have *practical applications* in morphologic studies of cortical development. Ontogenetic changes in the pattern of synapse distribution should be reflected in changes in the evoked potentials. Thus, by studying evoked potentials, we can select those gestational ages for morphologic study that are most likely to reveal functionally important changes in the distribution of synaptic contacts.

There is another, more technical use for the immature evoked potentials which we plan to incorporate in our future studies. Since individual deviations from normal development exist, those animals selected for morphologic analysis should be typical of the developmental age which they represent. The ontogenetic sequence of evoked potentials constitutes a scale for judging the cortical maturity of any individual animal. Evoked potentials can be easily obtained from many animals; in contrast, synapse distributions are laboriously determined in only a small number of animals. Therefore, before using a fetal animal for morphologic analysis, the evoked cortical surface response should be judged consistent with the normal pattern for that age (in respect to polarity and latency). Furthermore, the evoked potentials are extremely helpful in selecting the appropriate cortical region to be analyzed morphologically, since the fetal brain is relatively lissencephalic.

On the basis of the results obtained in the present study, we believe that the quantitative analysis of synapse distributions is a practical and meaningful approach to the study of developing cortical circuitry. Combined synaptoarchitectonic and cytoarchitectonic studies reveal two types of cortical layers which have different functional roles in neuronal circuitry. Neuronal perikarya plus their initial axon segments comprise a cytoarchitectonic layer, of which the prime functional characteristic is impulse origination. In terms of circuitry, a perikaryal layer is the *output zone* of a set of neurons. In contrast, the synaptic strata—regions of high synaptic density—are circumscribed loci in which impulses impinge upon the receptor zones of neurons. In terms of circuitry, a synaptic stratum is the *input zone* of a set of neurons, the perikarya of which may lie in different layers.

The perikaryal layers and the synaptic strata each produce different and characteristic electrophysiologic phenomena. The output from perikaryal layers is manifested by action potentials, which can be studied by the method of single unit analysis. In contrast, input to the dendrites (and somata) in a synaptic stratum is manifested by postsynaptic potentials.

The postsynaptic potentials of single neurons may be studied individually by intracellular recording, but that is especially difficult in young animals (Purpura, Shofer and Scarff, 1965). Postsynaptic activity in a set of neurons produces extracellular current flow which can be recorded from the cortical surface as a slow potential. Because of the distinctly stratified and relatively simple organization of synapses in immature cortex, the cortical surface potentials in young animals may be used to analyze postsynaptic activity in a specified set of neurons. Thus, it is possible, by means of cortical *surface* potentials alone, to study the functional maturation of specific intracortical neuronal elements.

The investigation reported in this paper is the first of a series of studies directed toward the elucidation of the ontogenesis of cortical circuitry. Future synaptoarchitectonic analyses of fetal cortex should permit us to locate the earliest synapses formed in cortex. The subsequent identification of pre- and postsynaptic elements would permit a comprehensive description of the neuronal circuits present at that age. Similar analyses at successive ontogenetic stages (in addition to the newborn which has been presented here) should reveal the continued formation of synapses and their role in cortical circuits of increasing complexity.

Summary

The establishment of cortical circuitry was studied by analyzing the spatial distribution of synapses in somesthetic cortex (SI) of neonatal dog. Relevant principles of cortical development are critically evaluated in a selective review of early and recent literature. A quantitative electron microscopic method was devised in order to analyze synaptic locations with respect to cytoarchitectonic layers of the cortex. It was demonstrated that synapses are not uniformly distributed through the cortex: strata of high synaptic density (synaptic strata) alternate with strata of low synaptic density. The synaptic strata have a definite relationship to cytoarchitectonic layers. Moreover, deep and superficial synapse-dense strata coincide with layers of precocious dendrite maturation. The synaptic strata are used to explain the polarity of evoked potentials characteristic of neonatal cortex. Both physiologic and morphologic data lead us to postulate that, in fetal life, the earliest synapses are established deep in the cortex. The functional significance of "synaptoarchitectonic" layers is compared with that of "cytoarchitectonic" layers. Principles relevant to a general formulation of developing cortical circuitry are discussed.

Acknowledgements. This work was supported by research grants from the U.S. Public Health Service, N.I.H. (NB 04012 and NB 08153) and by a special grant from the Joseph P. Kennedy, Jr., Memorial Foundation. Additional support was also obtained from N.I.C.H.D. Growth and Development Program, N.I.N.D.B. Grant NB 07935, and N.I.H. General Research Support to The Johns Hopkins University.

References[15]

Aghajanian, G. K., Bloom, F. E.: The formation of synaptic junctions in developing rat brain: a quantitative electron microscopic study. Brain Res. **6**, 716—727 (1967).

Amassian, V. E., Waller, H. J., Macy, Jr. J.,: Neural mechanisms of the primary somatosensory evoked potential. Ann. N. Y. Acad. Sci. **112**, 5—32 (1964).

Angevine Jun., J. B., Sidman, R. L.: Autoradiographic study of cell migration during histogenesis of cerebral cortex in the mouse. Nature (Lond.) **192**, 766—768 (1961).

Åström, K. E.: On the early development of the isocortex in fetal sheep. In: C. G. Bernhard and J. P. Schadé (eds.), Developmental neurology. Progress in brain research, vol. 26, p. 1—59. Amsterdam: Elsevier 1967.

Bernhard, C. G., Kolmodin, G. M., Meyerson, B. A.: On the prenatal development of function and structure in the somesthetic cortex of the sheep. In: C. G. Bernhard and J. P. Schadé (eds.), Developmental neurology. Progress in brain research, vol. 26, p. 60—77. Amsterdam: Elsevier 1967.

Bishop, G. H., Clare, M.: Sequence of events in optic cortex response to volleys of impulses in the radiation. J. Neurophysiol. **16**, 490—498 (1953).

Bloom, F. E., Aghajanian, G. K.: Cytochemistry of synapses: a selective staining method for electron microscopy. Science **154**, 1575—1577 (1966).

Brodal, A.: Neurological anatomy in relation to clinical medicine, 2nd ed. New York, etc.: Oxford University Press 1969.

Brodmann, K.: Vergleichende Lokalisationslehre der Großhirnrinde; in ihren Prinzipien dargestellt auf Grund des Zellenbaues. Leipzig: J. A. Barth 1909.

Bunge, M. B., Bunge, R. P., Peterson, E. R.: The onset of synapse formation in spinal cord cultures as studied by electron microscopy. Brain Res. **6**, 728—749 (1967).

Cajal, S. Ramón y: Sur la structure de l'écorce cérébrale de quelques mammifères. Cellule **7**, 123—176 (1891).

---

15 Multiple references in text appear in alphabetical order.

Cajal, S. Ramón y: Studien über die Hirnrinde des Menschen, H. 1, Die Sehrinde. Leipzig: J. A. Barth 1900.
— Studien über die Hirnrinde des Menschen, H. 5, Vergleichende Strukturbeschreibung und Histogenesis der Hirnrinde. Leipzig: J. A. Barth 1906.
— Histologie du système nerveux de l'homme et des vertébrés, tome II. Paris: Maloine 1911. [Ed. used by authors: Consejo Superior de Investigaciones Científicas, Madrid, 1955.]
Calvet, J., Calvet, M. C., Scherrer, J.: Étude stratigraphique corticale de l'activité EEG spontanée. Electroenceph. clin. Neurophysiol. **17**, 109—125 (1964).
Conel, J., Leroy: The postnatal development of the human cerebral cortex, vol. I, The cortex of the newborn. Cambridge, Mass.: Harvard University Press 1939.
Creutzfeldt, O. D., Watanabe, S., Lux, H. D.: Relations between EEG phenomena and potentials of single cortical cells. I. Evoked responses after thalamic and epicortical stimulation. Electroenceph. clin. Neurophysiol. **20**, 1—18 (1966).
Crosby, E. C., Humphrey, T., Lauer, E. W.: Correlative anatomy of the nervous system. New York: Macmillan 1962.
Eccles, J. C.: Interpretation of action potentials evoked in the cerebral cortex. Electroenceph. clin. Neurophysiol. **3**, 449—464 (1951).
Ellingson, R. J.: Cortical electrical responses to visual stimulation in the human infant. Electroenceph. clin. Neurophysiol. **12**, 663—677 (1960).
— Wilcott, R. C.: Development of evoked responses in visual and auditory cortices of kittens. J. Neurophysiol. **23**, 363—375 (1960).
Farber, D. A.: Evolution of specific evoked responses in visual cortex during ontogenesis. Neurosci. Transl. **6**, 651—657 (1968—69). [Transl. from Russian: Fiziol. Zh. (Mosk.) **54**, 778—786 (1968).]
Fox, M. W.: Neuronal development and ontogeny of evoked potentials in auditory and visual cortex of the dog. Electroenceph. clin. Neurophysiol. **24**, 213—226 (1968).
— Inman, O.: Persistence of Retzius-Cajal cells in developing dog brain. Brain Res. **3**, 192—194 (1966).
— — Himwich, W. A.: The postnatal development of neocortical neurons in the dog. J. comp. Neurol. **127**, 199—206 (1966).
Garma, L.: Ontogénèse des activités bio-électriques du cortex cerebral chez l'animal; leurs relations avec les états de veille et de sommeil. Paris: A. G. E. M. P. 1966.
Gay, H., Anderson, Th. F.: Serial sections for electron microscopy. Science **120**, 1071—1073 (1954).
Gray, E. G.: Axo-somatic and axo-dendritic synapses of the cerebral cortex: an electron microscopic study. J. Anat. (Lond.) **93**, 420—433 (1959).
Gruner, J. E., Zahnd, J. P.: Sur la maturation synaptique dans le cortex visuel du lapin. In: A. Minkowski (ed.), Regional development of the brain in early life, p. 125—133. Oxford: Blackwell 1967.
Hamuy, T. P., Bromiley, R. B., Woolsey, C. N.: Somatic afferent areas I and II of dog's cerebral cortex. J. Neurophysiol. **19**, 485—499 (1956).
Hubel, D. H., Wiesel, T. N.: Anatomical demonstration of columns in the monkey striate cortex. Nature (Lond.) **22**, 747—750 (1969).
Hunt, W. E., Goldring, S.: Maturation of evoked response of the visual cortex in the postnatal rabbit. Electroenceph. clin. Neurophysiol. **3**, 465—471 (1951).
Koelliker, A.: Handbuch der Gewebelehre des Menschen, Bd. 2, Nervensystem des Menschen und der Thiere, 6. Aufl. Leipzig: W. Engelmann 1896.
Landau, W. M., Clare, M. H.: A note on the characteristic response pattern in primary sensory projection cortex of the cat following a synchronous afferent volley. Electroenceph. clin. Neurophysiol. **8**, 457—464 (1956).
Lorente de Nó, R.: Studies on the structure of the cerebral cortex. J. Psychol. Neurol. (Lpz.) **45**, 381—438 (1933).
— Architectonics and structure of the cerebral cortex. In: J. F. Fulton, Physiology of the nervous system, p. 291—330. London etc.: Oxford University Press 1938.
Luft, J. H.: Improvements in epoxy resin embedding methods. J. biophys. biochem. Cytol. **9**, 409—414 (1961).

Marshall, W. H., Talbot, S. A., Ades, H. W.: Cortical response of the anesthetized cat to gross photic and electrical afferent stimulation. J. Neurophysiol. 6, 1—15 (1943).

Marty, R.: Développement post-natal des réponses sensorielles du cortex cérébral chez le chat et le lapin. Arch. Anat. micr. Morph. exp. 51, 129—264 (1962).

Meller, K., Breipohl, W., Glees, P.: The cytology of the developing molecular layer of mouse motor cortex. An electron microscopical and a Golgi impregnation study. Z. Zellforsch. 86, 171—183 (1968).

— — — Synaptic organization of the molecular and the outer granular layer in the motor cortex in the white mouse during postnatal development. A Golgi- and electronmicroscopical study. Z. Zellforsch. 92, 217—231 (1968).

Meyerson, B. A., Persson, H. E.: Evoked unitary and gross electric activity in the cerebral cortex in early prenatal ontogeny. Nature (Lond.) 221, 1248—1249 (1969).

Molliver, M. E.: An ontogenetic study of evoked somesthetic cortical responses in the sheep. In: C. G. Bernhard and J. P. Schadé (eds.), Developmental neurology. Progress in brain research, vol. 26, p. 78—91. Amsterdam: Elsevier 1967.

— Electrophysiologic parameters of ontogenesis in somesthetic cortex of fetal and neonatal dog. (Manuscript in preparation.)

— Van der Loos, H.: The synaptic strata of the somesthetic cortex in neonatal dog. Anat. Rec. 163, 317—318 (1969).

Mountcastle, V. B., Davies, Ph. W., Berman, A. L.: Response properties of neurons of cat's somatic sensory cortex to peripheral stimuli. J. Neurophysiol. 20, 374—407 (1957).

— Poggio, G. F.: Structural organization and general physiology of thalamotelencephalic systems. In: V. B. Mountcastle (ed.), Medical physiology, 12th ed., vol. II, p. 1277—1314. Saint Louis: Mosby 1968.

Nauta, W. J. H.: Terminal distribution of some afferent fiber systems in the cerebral cortex. Anat. Rec. 118, 333 (1954).

Noback, C. R., Purpura, D. P.: Postnatal ontogenesis of neurons in cat neocortex. J. comp. Neurol. 117, 291—307 (1961).

Oeconomos, D., Scherrer, J.: Étude des potentiels évoqués corticaux somesthésiques chez le chat nouveau-né. C. R. Soc. Biol. (Paris) 147, 1229—1232 (1953).

Perl, E. R., Whitlock, D. G.: Potentials evoked in cerebral somatosensory region. J. Neurophysiol. 18, 486—501 (1955).

Poljak, S. [= Polyak, S.]: An experimental study of the association, callosal, and projection fibers of the cerebral cortex of the cat. J. comp. Neurol. 44, 197—258 (1927).

Purpura, D. P.: Nature of electrocortical potentials and synaptic organizations in cerebral and cerebellar cortex. Int. Rev. Neurobiol. 1, 47—163 (1959).

— Analysis of axodendritic synaptic organizations in immature cerebral cortex. Ann. N. Y. Acad. Sci. 94, 604—654 (1961a).

— Ontogenetic analysis of some evoked synaptic activities in superficial neocortical neuropil. In: E. Florey (ed.), Nervous inhibition, p. 424—446. New York, etc.: Pergamon Press, Inc. 1961b.

— Carmichael, M. W., Housepian, E. M.: Physiological and anatomical studies of development of superficial axodendritic synaptic pathways in neocortex. Exp. Neurol. 2, 324—347 (1960).

— Shofer, R. J., Housepian, E. M., Noback, C. R.: Comparative ontogenesis of structure-function relations in cerebral and cerebellar cortex. In: D. P. Purpura and J. P. Schadé (eds.), Growth and maturation of the brain. Progress in brain research, vol. 4, p. 187—221. Amsterdam: Elsevier 1964.

— — Scarff, T.: Properties of synaptic activities and spike potentials of neurons in immature neocortex. J. Neurophysiol. 28, 925—942 (1965).

Rabinowicz, Th.: The cerebral cortex of the premature infant of the 8th month. In: D. P. Purpura and J. P. Schadé (eds), Growth and maturation of the brain. Progress in brain research, vol. 4, p. 39—92. Amsterdam: Elsevier 1964.

Retzius, G.: Ueber den Bau der Oberflächenschicht der Großhirnrinde beim Menschen und bei den Säugethieren. Verh. biol. Ver. (Stockh.) 3, 90—102 (1891).

— Die Cajal'schen Zellen der Großhirnrinde beim Menschen und bei Säugethieren. Biol. Unt. N. F. 5, 1—8 (1893).

Schadé, J. P., Van Groenigen, W. B.: Structural organization of the human cerebral cortex, 1, Maturation of the middle frontal gyrus. Acta anat. (Basel) **47**, 74—111 (1961).

Scheibel, M., Scheibel, A.: Some structural and functional substrates of development in young cats. In: W. A. Himwich and H. E. Himwich (eds.), The developing brain. Progress in brain research, vol. 9, p. 6—25. Amsterdam: Elsevier 1964.

Stefanowska, M.: Évolution des cellules nerveuses corticales chez la souris après la naissance. Trav. Lab. Physiol. Inst. Solvay **2**, 1—44 (1898).

Truex, R. C., Carpenter, M. B.: Strong and Elwyn's human neuroanatomy, 5th ed. Baltimore: Williams & Wilkins Co. 1964.

Van der Loos, H.: Dendro-dendritische verbindingen in de schors der grote hersenen. Haarlem, etc.: Stam 1959.

— Fine structure of synapses in the cerebral cortex. Z. Zellforsch. **60**, 815—825 (1963).

— Anatomic and physiologic considerations. Chap. 120 of Sect. 16: Regulating systems — Neural. In: R. E. Cooke (ed.), The biologic basis of pediatric practice, p. 1177—1200. New York: McGraw-Hill 1968.

— A versatile variation of Golgi's method. (Manuscript in preparation.)

Venable, J. H., Coggeshall, R.: A simplified lead citrate stain for use in electron microscopy. J. Cell Biol. **25**, 407—408 (1965).

Verley, R.: Recherches sur le développement des activités électro-corticales avec des électrodes corticales radiaires. J. Physiol. (Paris) **57**, 407—436 (1965).

Vignal, W.: Recherches sur le développement de la substance corticale du cerveau et du cervelet. Arch. Physiol. norm. path. (Paris), Ser. IV, **2**, 311—338 (1888).

Voeller, K., Pappas, G. D., Purpura, D. P.: Electron microscopic study of development of cat superficial neocortex. Exp. Neurol. **7**, 107—130 (1963).

Index